GOD AND THE EMBRYO
RELIGIOUS VOICES ON
STEM CELLS AND CLONING

Brent Waters

and

Ronald Cole-Turner

Editors

GEORGETOWN UNIVERSITY PRESS
WASHINGTON, D.C.

Georgetown University Press, Washington, D.C.
© 2003 by Georgetown University Press. All rights reserved.
Printed in the United States of America.

10 9 8 7 6 5 4 3 2   2003

This book is printed on acid-free recycled paper meeting the requirements of the
American National Standard for Permanence in Paper for Printed Library Materials.

Library of Congress Cataloging-in-Publication Data

God and the embryo : religious voices on stem cells and cloning /
Brent Waters and Ronald Cole-Turner, editors.
        p. cm
Includes bibliographical references and index.
    ISBN 0-87840-998-X (pbk. : alk. paper)
    1. Human cloning—Religious aspects. 2. Stem cells—Research—Religious aspects.
I. Waters, Brent. II. Cole-Turner, Ronald, 1948–
    QH442.2.G63 2003
    241'.64957—dc21

                                                        2003006470

Contents

Appendices

Acknowledgments

This book began in public presentations made by several of its contributors at the research colloquy "The Ethics of Human Embryonic Stem Cell Research," cosponsored by the Center for Ethics and Values and *Science and Spirit* magazine and held at Garrett-Evangelical Theological Seminary, in Evanston, Illinois, in October 2001, and at a panel discussion sponsored by the Pew Forum on Religion and Public Life titled "The Moral Status of the Embryo," held at the National Press Club in Washington, D.C., in February 2002. We acknowledge with gratitude the role of both these events in helping us develop the plan for this book.

Chapter 3, by Gene Outka, originally appeared as "The Ethics of Human Stem Cell Research," in the *Kennedy Institute of Ethics Journal* 12:2 (2002), 175–213. © The Johns Hopkins University Press. Reprinted with permission of The Johns Hopkins University Press.

We appreciate the kindness of several organizations that gave us permission to reprint their material in the appendices. We express our appreciation to the Holy Synod of Bishops of the Orthodox Church in America for permission to reprint its "Embryonic Stem Cell Research in the Perspective of Orthodox Christianity: A Statement of the Holy Synod of Bishops of the Orthodox Church in America"; to the Presbyterian Church (USA) for permission to reprint "Overture 01-50. On Adopting a Resolution Enunciating Ethical Guidelines for Fetal Tissue and Stem Cell Research—From the Presbytery of Baltimore"; to the Executive Committee of the Southern Baptist

Convention for permission to reprint "Resolution: On Human Embryonic and Stem Cell Research," which was approved by the messengers to the Southern Baptist Convention, 16 June 1999; to the United Methodist Church for permission to reprint its statement, "Urgent Action Alert: Urge Senators to Support Complete Ban on Human Cloning," which includes materials from *The Book of Resolutions of the United Methodist Church* © 2000 by The United Methodist Publishing House (used by permission); to the United Church of Christ for permission to reprint its General Synod resolution, "Support for Federally Funded Research on Embryonic Stem Cells" of July 2001; to *Ethics and Medicine: An International Journal of Bioethics* for "A Theologian's Brief on the Place of the Human Embryo within the Christian Tradition, and the Theological Principles for Evaluating Its Moral Status," which appeared in the fall 2001 (17:3) issue; and to the Union of Orthodox Jewish Congregations of America and the Rabbinical Council of America for their joint statement "Cloning Research, Jewish Tradition and Public Policy."

Introduction

RONALD COLE-TURNER

The creation of the first human embryos by cloning was announced late in 2001 by a group of researchers working for a private corporation, Advanced Cell Technologies (ACT), of Worcester, Massachusetts.[1] The work was done in order to determine whether it is possible to create cloned embryos from which to harvest embryonic stem cells. Advocates of this goal, sometimes called "therapeutic cloning," believe it holds the key to successful treatment for a wide range of diseases, from Parkinson's disease to diabetes, that currently claim the lives of as many as 3,000 Americans every day.

What was disturbing to many about this research is that ACT set out on this pathway on its own, accountable only to itself and its investors. Human cloning, including therapeutic human cloning that produces no baby, is controversial, to put it mildly. Nearly everyone on both sides of the controversy acknowledges that human cloning is a milestone of sorts in human history. That a private corporation would cross the threshold into the age of cloning, as if it were nothing but a corporate strategy or a mere line in its R&D budget, is troubling.

To be fair, however, we must recognize that ACT broke no laws, nor did the company fail in any duty to obtain permission for its work. In fact, on scientific grounds alone, the researchers' publication was premature but perhaps commendable because it provided some public account of their work.

Furthermore, the legal and moral context in which ACT does its work is hardly the company's fault. The responsibility in fact lies with our political leadership and even more fundamentally with the role played by religion in the American political context. Because of the intensity with which religious groups have struggled in the past over abortion, and because of the link between that debate and the question of the human embryo, intense religious conflicts over the status of the embryo and the legitimacy of embryo research have helped create a political stalemate. As a result, the federal government does not fund any embryo research, but it does not prevent it either. Publicly funded researchers, who are held to high standards of public accountability, cannot conduct this work in the United States. Privately funded researchers, with almost no legal constraints, however, can pursue this work at will.

The contributors to this volume represent these sharp religious conflicts. When it comes to the legitimacy of embryo research, we agree on nothing. We do believe, however, that religious disagreement should not keep us from respecting each other, talking to each other, or hoping to persuade each other. That we seek to do so here in print is evidence of our belief that through greater religious understanding will come better ethics and better policy. In the broadest terms, our hope is to contribute to a discussion that improves U.S. and global policy, even though we disagree for now on what would count as improvement.

In part I, "Frameworks," we begin to explore the issues. My essay introduces the subject and invites the reader to join the debate. Brent Waters challenges us to broaden our understanding of "public" and therefore of the role that religion plays in an enriched and multifaceted public argument. Gene Outka's article surveys the often-unexamined assumptions the underlie the debate and then proposes a new way to argue for a position somewhere in the "middle."

Part II turns to the central question of the embryo, first with an examination by Brent Waters of the various arguments about the status of the embryo, which he follows by posing the question, "Is the embryo my neighbor?" James Peterson takes on the question of the personhood of the embryo, arguing that traditional theological method does *not* lead to the view that personhood begins at conception. My essay, "Principles and Politics," reflects on the reasons for this conflict especially among Christians and argues for the benefits of a pragmatic agreement in the absence of the ever-elusive theological consensus. Robert Song, who writes out of his context in England and thus of laws in the United Kingdom that permit embryo research, offers a vigorous argument about the "benefit of the doubt" that should be accorded to the embryo.

Finally, in part III, "Research," we consider some of the principles that govern research policy. Ted Peters and Gaymon Bennett propose that beneficence, or the prospect of doing good for those affected by diseases possibly treatable by embryonic stem cells, is the preeminent religious value in the debate. Kevin FitzGerald, S.J., drawing on his work in medical research and in moral theology to show the complexity of the issues and the ambiguity of many of the terms in the debate, counters by questioning whether embryo research is really necessary to help those in need. Laurie Zoloth draws on the textual tradition of Judaism and invites us to stand back for a moment from the immediate concerns of embryo research policy to reflect on our place as human moral agents in a physically imperfect world. Finally, Sondra Wheeler concludes the volume with an appeal first for precision but most of all for explicit theological grounding for our conversation. For indeed, it is only as people of faith, whose lives and words are nurtured by living traditions, that we who speak here have anything to say.

Note

1. Jose B. Cibelli, Ann A. Kiessling, Kerrianne Cunniff, Charlotte Richards, Robert P. Lanza, and Michael D. West, "Somatic Cell Nuclear Transfer in Humans: Pronuclear and Early Embryonic Development," *e-biomed: The Journal of Regenerative Medicine* 2 (2001): 25–31.

PART ONE

Frameworks

ONE

Religion Meets Research

RONALD COLE-TURNER

I s it ever right to use the human embryo as a tool of research or therapy? Few questions have divided us so deeply. On one side are the many
Christians who look at the embryo and see a member of the human family,
a neighbor, a being that is human and worthy of the same protection as any
of us all the more so because it is tiny and vulnerable. On the other side of
the debate are the many Christians and most Jews who see the human embryo not as another human person but as a cell with the extraordinary potential to divide and develop into a person, and therefore of less value in its
present state than, say, a baby.

This impasse over the embryo affects scientific research and the future of
medicine, determining how and where research is done, who approves it, who
might benefit, and what the long-term implications might be. The impasse
is mediated through the political arena, and in the United States, at least, political leaders are unable to agree on policy. But beneath the science and the
politics, the impasse is religious, grounded in two competing views of the
dignity of the embryo.

When they have no need for clarity, religious traditions have a high degree of tolerance for differences of opinion and for ambiguity of viewpoint
among their followers. But when it becomes necessary to clear things up, as
it is now regarding the embryo, ambiguity is flushed out of its shadows into
the full light of cross-examination, clarity is demanded, and tolerance suffers.
We see this happening today in regard to how religious people and institutions

look at the human embryo. Everyone has an opinion, it seems, and no one likes anyone else's opinion.

In simpler times, so little was known scientifically about the nature of pre-natal life, and so little could be done about it in any case, that religious people felt no need to have an opinion, much less choose sides. There was, of course, a general religious attitude of respect for nascent life and of doing what little could be done to nourish and protect it, as well as general opposition to abor-tion, but there was no dogma or required unity of opinion about its status or condition.

This is changing, first because of advances in scientific understanding of embryology that reveal to us in great detail the stunning complexity of the genetic and cellular processes through which the embryo passes from its for-mation in fertilization to its development into the fetus and the newborn. These developments evoke religious wonder and summon a theological re-sponse. But perhaps more important are the developments in biomedical technology, which rest on the science but go far beyond it in forcing us to make up our minds. The birth of the world's first in vitro child in 1978 ush-ered in an era in which we relocated the embryo so that it may be created outside the body and exist, at least for a short time, out where we can see it and get at it with all our tests and probes and manipulative instruments. Thus, technology changes reality and requires a decision: is it right to create an em-bryo outside the body, to store it, to discard it, or to donate it to another cou-ple? What sort of thing is this embryo that we have made, that we should or should not do these things to it? Does its location or the manner of its cre-ation affect what it is or what we owe it?

More recent advances in the technology of the embryo have now forced us to ask still more pointed questions and come to more sharply divided opinions, so much so that religious people now take stands against each other in public over the meaning and the morals of the embryo. The announce-ment of the birth of Dolly the cloned sheep now means that it is possible to create mammalian embryos, not just by conception (either in vivo or in vitro) but by a process known as somatic cell nuclear transfer (SCNT).[1] Human embryos may be created, not just through the joining of sperm and egg to form a novel genetic combination, not in other words by fertilization, but by the transfer into an egg of the nuclear genetic material sucked from a cell of an adult.

Is this technological concoction still an embryo? Most of us agree that it is an embryo of sorts, at least in its presumed potential to form a new life, and that it is probably due the same respect as an embryo created by other means. But we wonder how it differs from embryos that come from fertilization and whether that difference in the technology of its origin amounts to a moral and ontological distinction about its dignity. If anything, the cloned embryo seems to have far less likelihood or potential than the fertilized embryo to actually become a human being, because of the subtleties of genetic signaling that take place when an embryo is created by fertilization but not when one is created by cloning. So anyone who believes that an embryo is valuable primarily because of its potential to become a person has to contend with the fact that the cloned embryo most likely has less potential. But still we somehow sense that it is an embryo, if for no other reason than because we have no other category in which to put it.

Another recent advance of equal importance for our discussion lies in the area of stem cells. In 1998, scientists reported on their work in isolating human embryonic stem cells.[2] As the name suggests, these cells are derived from embryos, which were destroyed in the process. The original work was done using spare embryos donated by couples who had created them in reproductive clinics. The attraction of embryonic stem cells is that they seem capable of developing into any other type of cell in the human body. That means they could be implanted in the body to replace cells that are damaged by injury or illness, thereby helping the patient's own body to regenerate tissues and organs, possibly including brain regions or the spinal cord. Another attraction of embryonic stem cells is that they seem capable of being grown indefinitely in the laboratory. That is, under the right conditions, they divide indefinitely without losing their other characteristics.

There are other types of stem cells, usually referred to as "adult stem cells," meaning that they are derived from something other than an embryo. They seem to have somewhat less ability than embryonic stem cells to develop into any type of cell in the body, but that is unclear for now.[3] Most scientists working in this field favor support for research into both types of stem cells, adult and embryonic, in order to advance the whole field together.

One problem that stands in the way of using embryonic stem cells in medicine is that these cells will most likely trigger an immune response when they are implanted in a patient. To minimize that response, researchers hope to develop many stem cell lines and then choose the right one for each patient, in the hope of ensuring the lowest level of immune response. Even so, immunosuppression drugs will need to be used, and their use clouds the potential of this therapy. A possible alternative approach is to combine cloning or SCNT with embryonic stem cell technology. For each patient, physicians could use cloning to create an embryo that matches the patient's DNA. The embryo would be destroyed after a few days of cultivation, and the stem cells would be harvested, cultured, and implanted in the patient, whose immune system would recognize them as the body's own cells. The problem, of course, is that creating and destroying an embryo would be a necessary part of stem cell therapy, at least for some patients. For some patients, the choice may literally come down to their morals or their health, either consent against principle to an embryo being created and destroyed for therapy or go untreated. In that regard, the most trouble-free approach, if ever feasible, would be to harvest adult stem cells from the patient's own body, cultivate them, and return them to the body. Some scientists think that, if they are allowed to pursue embryonic stem cell research at this stage, they may someday discover how to avoid using embryos altogether. It is probably true that most patients, even if they objected to the destruction of embryos to develop the technology in the first place, would accept treatments that did not involve destroying any more embryos.

Combining cloning or SCNT with embryonic stem cell technology, as we just described, is sometimes referred to as "therapeutic" cloning. No one has yet proven that there is any therapy here, so it would probably be more accurate to speak of it as nonreproductive cloning, in order to distinguish it from reproductive cloning, which intends to produce a baby. This distinction between reproductive and nonreproductive cloning is critical for understanding the debates over cloning policy. Nearly everyone is opposed to reproductive cloning, if for no other reason than the risks involved, and so every piece of legislation that is introduced and every policy position that is offered includes either a temporary moratorium or a permanent ban on reproductive cloning.[4] The debate, whether in terms of public policy or religious morality, is not over what we should do, at least for now, about reproductive cloning but whether we should permit nonreproductive cloning, specifically the creation of human embryos through SCNT for the purposes of research or therapy.

So far, most Christian statements addressing this question have opposed nonreproductive cloning and embryo research. A few statements of Christian churches, as well as the strong majority view among Jewish statements, have been open to the legitimacy of nonreproductive cloning and other forms of embryo research.[5] Bills have been introduced in the U.S. Congress both permitting and prohibiting nonreproductive cloning. As of the summer of 2002, the majority of the members of the U.S. House of Representatives supports prohibition, while the majority in the U.S. Senate (including leading members of both political parties) favors permitting nonreproductive cloning and limited embryo research. President George W. Bush opposes this research, at least when it comes to federal funds being available to support it, but he has left open a window that permits federal funds for research on embryonic stem cells derived prior to the date he announced his policy, August 9, 2001.

Technology and Morals

As we consider these developments in research and in science policy, we should remind ourselves that, although science offers us new ways to understand nature, technology confronts us with something far more puzzling and provocative. Science helps us see things in new ways, often at the expense of old ways, but technology offers up new things to see, new entities and new relationships between familiar entities. Consider the cloned embryo created through nuclear transfer. Never before has such a thing existed, not even through twinning. We do not know what we think about it now because we have never had to before. But consider also the possibility that in the future, human embryonic stem cells themselves could be turned into human embryos. Would they be regarded as the moral equivalent of embryos, and would we have to regard their antecedents—the stem cells themselves—as potential embryos and therefore as potential persons? When we juxtapose technology and morals, as we must, we should learn to expect that technology will stretch, and often break, the categories of thought that previously defined our moral view. Technology forces us to deal with realities that have never before existed, and we can only imagine what lies ahead in the technologies of human biomedical self-modification and what new and bizarre forms of humanity we will have to try to understand, as we human beings modify our biological nature and combine it with elements from other species or from computers.

Even more subtle is the way that technology restructures relationships. The embryo, whether cloned or from in vitro fertilization, is now out in front of us, in a dish and vulnerable. When it is placed in front of us as an object, it belongs no longer to the mysterious processes of life or to the woman whose body nourishes it in hiding, but to the laboratory that created it, to researchers who hope to open its secrets and, when they are through, discard it, as they seem to have a right to do. Even if the embryo is created by an infertile couple at a reproductive clinic, it is probably one of many, which may or may not be chosen. If it is not chosen, it may then be stored in liquid nitrogen, destroyed, or perhaps donated for research. We can take all these as new forms of action with embryos because technology has put the embryo before us, redefining its physical location and its moral relationship to those to whom it belongs, and so making it an object of knowledge, purpose, and will.

All this is sobering enough at the scale of one embryo, but by putting the embryo in front of us, these processes place human nature itself before us and make the future of our species into a project. For, if we modify ourselves, not just through reproductive cloning but through the far more significant step of human germ line modification (so called "designer babies"), it will most likely be possible because of the embryo's physical relation to us and in fact because the embryo itself is the first object of these interventions.[6] We simply do not know what lies ahead in terms of the technologies of the embryo. The most recent discoveries coming from the Human Genome Project suggest that our ability to modify genes may not lead as automatically as we once thought to the ability to control or modify traits. The relationship between genes and traits is complex and subtle, to put it mildly, and the power to edit a DNA sequence must never be confused with the power to design traits. Nevertheless, as we learn more about these very subtleties of nature and acquire other technologies of cell modification, it is clear that human nature will be rendered increasingly pliable in our hands and malleable by our technology.

In the long term, what might this mean? Some have suggested that the combination of access to the embryo and the technologies of biological modification will mean that we will soon become the engineers of our own evolution. Other technologies will also play a role here, such as information technology and its linkage to the human brain through direct electrode-neuron connections. No one knows how far this will go, or if in time we will recreate ourselves in the image of our own yearnings for greater intellect, more durable health, and longer life. The key point to recognize, however, is that the technologies of embryo manipulation will play a central role in whatever pathway we take toward this future of human self-modification. For this reason, the question of the embryo looms before us, not merely as a question about a tiny cluster of cells or as the political impasse of the year but as nothing less than the question of the future of the species. Embryo modification will become species modification, with the embryo as the point of access.

If that is correct, we can see why it is necessary for us to come to a moral understanding of the technologies of the embryo and to a political capacity to guide their use. If we fail to understand and guide today's technologies, we will have little chance of success when we face, as we soon shall, the far greater challenge of understanding and guiding the technologies of human modification, human enhancement, and human transformation. The pathway to these audacious technologies passes through today's embryo research, and we must learn now to understand, guide, and direct this research if we are to guide our own future.

Religion and Public Policy

The embryo is key both to the technology and to the formation of public policy. If embryo modification will become species modification with the embryo as the point of access, embryo research policy will become the groundwork through which we create a public, deliberative, and participatory context to guide the development and use of the technologies that change us.

A particular burden in this regard faces the United States. Failure in the United States to develop a federal policy on embryo research will mean that research will proceed anyway with private funding and without public accountability. Other countries will be discouraged from developing their own policy, for fear that researchers will prefer the uncontrolled U.S. environment to even minimal levels of public accountability elsewhere.

On these matters—why regulation is needed, how it is possible, and why the United States plays a special role here—a persuasive argument has been offered by Francis Fukuyama. The weakness of Fukuyama's case, however, lies in overlooking the role of religion. He summarizes his argument this way: "Putting these facts together—that an embryo has a moral status somewhere between that of an infant and that of other types of cells and tissues, and that the transformation of the embryo into something with a higher status is a mysterious process—suggest that if we are to do things like harvest stem cells from embryos, we should put a lot of limits and constraints around this activity to make sure that it does not become a precedent for other uses of the unborn that would push the envelop further."[7]

For many people of religious conviction, however, the question of the embryo is not simply a matter of "putting these facts together." Religious convictions and apprehensions bear down on this tiny dot, the embryo, as a focal

point for profound concerns about human identity, dignity, and manipula-
bility. These intensely religious concerns mean the embryo is politically
charged, and any analysis of public policy must take religion into account.
The highly charged religious context lies directly behind our failure so far in
the United States to develop a policy and a regulatory framework for embryo research. Other factors, such as the antiregulatory sentiment of the moment, surely play a role, but the reason for our failure lies finally in our conflicted views about the embryo, and nowhere is the conflict more sharp or
intense than among religious people, Christians in particular.

We should not expect this debate to end any time soon, but it may be possible—indeed, this is the hope of those of us who contribute to this volume—
to arrive at greater mutual understanding and respect, to attain greater clarity in details of our positions, and to find more common ground than perhaps
we imagined. Furthermore, we want to set out our arguments for the wider
public, who have a right to know what religious beliefs bear on public policy, why they are so strongly held, and what prospects there are for finding a
way forward. Finally, we offer these essays to those in our own various traditions within Christianity and Judaism in the hope that we will come to
clearer understandings of what they affirm and, perhaps more important, what
they do not.

In so doing we hope to clear up several misperceptions. Perhaps the simplest and most obvious misperception is that the debate over the embryo is
merely today's battle in the perennial war between religion and science. The
"war" itself turns out to be a myth based on sloppy history, as historians of
science have now shown, and the notion of a conflict between religion and
science over the embryo turns out to be an equally simplistic and inaccurate
view of what is going on. Religious people are divided on the issue, which
means first of all that if there is conflict, it is religion versus religion, not religion versus science. But more important, if there is anything that the religious participants in this debate agree on, it is that they all are promedicine
and proscience, strongly supporting the advances in scientific understanding
and the medical technologies that come in their wake. There are people, of
course, who oppose technology wholesale, but almost without exception these
are not religious people or at least religious leaders and scholars in the major
faith traditions. Nevertheless, too many news reports still claim (and too many
scientists still believe) that the embryo debate is religion battling science.

Another misperception is that the views of religious people are simple,
one-dimensional, dogmatic, or based on claims of special knowledge. Any serious reader of these essays will find complexity and subtlety of argument

mixed with confessions of uncertainty and indecision. No one here believes that the embryo is merely a bunch of cells, nor does anyone believe that the embryo is simply a person in the same sense that you and I are persons. All the positions taken here lie in between these simplistic extremes. They occupy various points on the continuum of the degree of respect we owe embryos. For some of us, the embryo should be treated as if it is a person even if we do not claim certain knowledge that it is a person, and we demand for it special care because of its weakness and vulnerability. For others, myself included, the embryo is something less than that, but not nothing and not to be treated without concern for its worth.

Another misconception is that religious positions on embryo research are nothing more than an extension of positions taken in the abortion debate. Of course, there is some correspondence between the two, as there should be. Religious bodies that defend a position of choice in abortion are the only ones that defend the possibility of embryo research, but the inverse relationship does not hold. That is, some churches, perhaps most notably the United Methodist Church, defend choice in abortion but oppose embryo research. At first glance, we could say this is a matter of institutional inconsistency, as if one part of a large organization does not know or feel constrained by what another part does or thinks. But the issue is more complex than that, and its explanation lies in the development of church doctrine and policy over the past thirty years, during which there has been a steady movement toward more conservative positions on these issues. Positions on abortion previously taken are not easily abandoned, but the new questions posed by embryo research prompt churches to articulate new positions that are not necessarily consistent with what went before, but perhaps reflect the changed theological consciousness of the church. The tangled relationship between the questions of abortion and of embryo research is too complex for simple consistency.

Perhaps even more puzzling is how positions on embryo research reflect positions on in vitro fertilization. One might reasonably expect that anyone who permits couples to create multiple embryos for reproductive purposes, and in so doing to store and perhaps destroy some embryos, might also permit scientists to create embryos for research, or at least to use some of the embryos unneeded for reproductive purposes, embryos that may otherwise be destroyed. Not everyone is so logical, though, perhaps because they place a greater value on reproductive than scientific freedom.

All this is worth noting because we do, in fact, live in a culture that tolerates considerable inconsistency in these matters. We allow abortion for nearly any purpose, and we allow couples to pay reproductive clinics to create embryos and then destroy them if they are unwanted, but we do not want to sanction the freedom of scientists to create embryos for research or for possible therapy. In doing so, we have created an incoherent body of policies that permits abortion, privatizes and thereby ignores in vitro fertilization, prohibits public funding for embryo research and thereby avoids any federal role in overseeing it, but permits privately funded research to do whatever it wants.

All these inconsistencies and conflicts are found in the faith traditions themselves, not just between traditions, but also among adherents of single traditions. Many religious organizations have endorsed some version of choice in abortion, or there is some sizeable group within the tradition that has done so. Many have accepted in vitro fertilization without comment, allowing their members to choose it almost as if faith played no role in the decision, but many of them balk at the idea of scientists creating embryos, or at least they cannot bring themselves to permit this publicly, even though they permit much more to infertile couples or pregnant women. When religion permits the choice of abortion or the choice of in vitro fertilization but forbids or is silent on embryo research, one must forgive scientists who think that religion is antiscience.

If, however, religion is to understand its own convictions about the embryo and explain them to a wider audience, its adherents must ask how they know about the embryo at all. In the language of theologians, this is a question about theological method. By what method of religious knowing can we say that we know how we are to regard the embryo with respect to its most profound meaning, with respect to its humanity and its imaging of its Creator, or with respect to its claim on the dignity of human life in relationship to God? We can, of course, learn from the science of embryology, and we can (as we surely must) take into account all the technologies of embryo creation and manipulation. But what is it that theology knows that science per se does not know? And how does theology know it?

The answer that theologians are trained to give is that we turn to scripture and tradition and bring them into some sort of dialogue or interaction with other sources of knowledge, including the sciences. We do so until we have achieved a new level of insight that respects science or other secular sources but is not limited to them, going on instead to propose additional claims that are intimated if not spelled out by ancient texts and authorities and by the general conviction of the faithful. That is the official answer, but, in fact, we simply do not agree on, or even know, how we know. Underlying our disagreements about embryo policy are disagreements about embryo theology, and underlying these are disagreements about theological method.

Finding agreement on theological method is not likely, certainly not in this volume, but noting the problem highlights our difficulty. The religious impasse over the embryo, which so greatly impairs our political capacity to guide today's research or tomorrow's applications, is not easily resolved because we disagree about why we disagree. We all read the same science and the same scriptures, but we put them together with different formulas and different claims of authority for each. We all believe human life and human action are to be offered in obedience and praise to the same God, but we have profoundly different understandings of what God is doing in our time and requiring us to do.

So we offer our opinions with humility and respect for each other, but also with that boldness of constructive imagination required of anyone who ventures beyond the familiar and into the unknown. Never before has it been quite so obvious that ideas have consequences, most of all ideas about God and humanity and embryos. What we think is what we will do, and what we will do is what we shall become.

Notes

1. I. Wilmut, A. E. Schnieke, J. McWhir, A. J. Kind, and K. H. Campbell, "Viable Off-spring Derived from Fetal and Adult Mammalian Cells," *Nature* 385 (1997): 810–13 [erratum in *Nature* 386 (1997): 200].

2. J. A. Thomson, J. Itskovitz-Eldor, S. S. Shapiro, M. A. Waknitz, J. J. Swiergiel, V. S. Marshall, and J. M. Jones, "Embryonic Stem Cell Lines Derived from Human Blastocysts," *Science* 282 (1998): 1145–57 [erratum in *Science* 282 (1998): 1827]. Similar cells were derived from aborted fetuses, reported by M. J. Shamblott, J. Axelman, S. Wang, E. M. Bugg, J. W. Littlefield, P. J. Donovan, P. D. Blumenthal, G. R. Huggins, and J. D. Gearhart in "Derivation of Pluripotent Stem Cells from Cultured Human Primordial Germ Cells," *Proceedings of the National Academy of Sciences USA* 95 (1998): 13726–31 [erratum in *Proceedings of the National Academy of Sciences USA* 96 (1999): 1162].

3. For a highly promising report of the versatility of adult-derived stem cells, see Yuehua Jiang, Balkrishna N. Jahagirdar, R. Lee Reinhardt, Robert E. Schwartz, C. Dirk Keenek, Xilma R. Ortiz-Gonzalezk, Morayma Reyes, Todd Lenvik, Troy Lund, Mark Blackstad, Jingbo Du, Sara Aldrich, Aaron Lisberg, Walter C. Lowk, David A. Largaespada, and Catherine M. Verfaillie, "Pluripotency of Mesenchymal Stem Cells Derived from Adult Marrow," *Nature* 27 (June 2002): 41–49.

4. For religious responses to reproductive cloning, see Ronald Cole-Turner, ed., *Human Cloning: Religious Responses* (Louisville, Ky.: Westminster/John Knox Press, 1997), and *Beyond Cloning: Religion and the Remaking of Humanity* (Harrisburg, Pa.: Trinity Press International, 2001).

5. For these texts, see appendices.

6. There are several ways in which human germ line modification could be achieved, but most agree that any full-scale attempt at human modification or enhancement would no doubt depend on our ability to work directly on the embryo. For a full discussion, see Audrey R. Chapman and Mark S. Frankel, *Designing Our Descendants: The Promises and Perils of Genetic Modification* (Baltimore: American Association for the Advancement of Science and Johns Hopkins University Press, 2003).

7. Francis Fukuyama, *Our Posthuman Future: Consequences of the Biotechnology Revolution* (New York: Farrar, Straus, and Giroux, 2002), 176–77.

TWO

What Is the Appropriate Contribution of Religious Communities in the Public Debate on Embryonic Stem Cell Research?

BRENT WATERS

The most important word in the question posed by the title of this chapter is "appropriate," for it implies that religious traditions and communities are capable of making inappropriate contributions to the public debate on embryonic stem cell research. Admittedly, there is historical evidence to justify this fear, particularly with respect to religious commentary on scientific issues that is often ill informed. Yet before we can identify the difference between what is an appropriate and inappropriate contribution, we must first define what we mean by "public" and describe what kind of debate we should be endeavoring to undertake.

The Public Context and Religious Contributions to Public Moral Discourse

What is "public" is *not* restricted to legislation, legal jurisdiction, or activities conducted or funded by governmental agencies. This would mean accepting a very narrow understanding of what is public (as well as what the public is), thereby constraining both the breadth and depth of the debate over the morality of embryonic stem cell research. Rather, the public is comprised of a highly complex nexus of social spheres or human associations. These associations may be voluntary or nonvoluntary, relatively large or small, formal or informal, highly institutionalized or loosely knit together. Some of these associations may be self-contained, whereas others are closely related.

Moreover, virtually every individual lives in a series of these overlapping associations. For instance, we are simultaneously members of families, workers, churchgoers, volunteers, and citizens, and who we are, particularly as members of the public, cannot be reduced to any one of these roles.

I present this image of a series of human associations or social spheres to emphasize that public life (and the life of the public) is not simply a relationship between the state and individual citizens. Instead, relationships and institutions comprising civil society mediate it. It is within and among such associations as families, religious communities, charitable organizations, corporations and the like (associations that in the United States have oddly come to be perceived as "private") that virtues and values are formed that either serve us well or badly in forming the contours of our common, public life. We learn how to form, navigate, and maintain the fabric of public life largely in our daily interactions with our families, coworkers, neighbors, friends, and strangers, and not simply in resolving controversial political issues or addressing thorny policy questions. To be a public means that we share bonds of relationships and affinities that are given and largely not of our choosing.

Consequently, there are two appropriate contributions that religious communities can offer to the public debate on embryonic stem cell research. First, religious communities should keep in mind and remind others of the larger and more expansive public context in which this debate over embryonic stem cell research is being waged. Admittedly, this debate will be conducted largely with legislators, government agencies, and the courts in mind. Enacting suitable legislation, establishing just policies, and setting legal precedents are important tasks, and religious communities (as well as individuals motivated by religious faith) certainly have a right to try to influence the course and outcomes of these political and legal processes. There is much at stake in the laws, policies, and procedures that will delineate and govern this research.

But this is not the only venue in which this debate can or should be conducted. It is not only laws, policies, and procedures that will affect us. In addition, the very manner in which this debate is pursued will have a formative influence on the human associations comprising civil society, as well as our very perception of what it means to be a public. The rhetoric we employ, for example, to describe what an embryo is and what it is not, or how it is related or not related to larger human communities, will shape our perceptions of the relative strength or weakness of the biological bonds that bind us together *as a* people, as well as the moral duties and obligations accompanying that affinity. It does make a difference if we come to perceive (at least some) embryos as being more akin to property that can be used, exchanged, or otherwise developed for purposes unrelated to procreation, as opposed to perceiving embryos as in some sense already related to or a part of the human communities that create them.

Again, I want to be clear: I am not suggesting that issues concerning legislation, policies, and funding are trivial or unimportant, but the largely procedural rhetoric these activities tend to promote cannot provide an adequate basis for public moral debate that the gravity of embryonic stem cell research requires. Perhaps the most important role religious communities can play in this debate is to mine and refine the deep resources of their theological and moral resources, in order to craft richer vocabularies that take into account a more expansive vision of the life of the public to describe what we are endeavoring to do and what foreseen and unforeseen consequences we might encounter in the research now envisioned. In this respect, religious communities can offer alternative accounts of what binds together human communities other than a thinly conceived social contract (which is itself haunted by an unhappy history of exclusion rather than inclusion) that can all too easily and expediently rebuff something like an embryo as an irrelevant consideration in pursuing health care goals and objectives.

The second appropriate contribution religious communities can offer is to express in as clear and forthright a manner as possible the principal beliefs, convictions, and claims that inform their moral assessments of embryonic stem cell research. I realize that I am contradicting the conventional wisdom of our day, which insists that it is precisely these larger and divisive declarations that need to be excluded from the public arena. As Albert Jonsen and Stephen Toulmin contend, turning to "matters of principle" stifles public moral debate on highly controversial issues. We are better off concentrating on specific objectives and fair procedures for achieving them. Our only hope for attaining some semblance of "moral certitude" in the public arena is to focus on practical considerations or judgments. According to Jonsen and Toulmin consensus on practical details can often be achieved by individuals holding highly disparate values so long as the reasons for prompting such agreements remain unknown. It is only when moral debate soars to the "level of principles" that individuals inevitably go their "separate ways." By encouraging religious communities to express their normative beliefs and convictions openly, we are submitting ourselves to a "tyranny of principles" because we will become bogged down in interminable and irresolvable debates over such contentious issues as when life begins or when is personhood present. Individuals are, of course, free to hold whatever private opinions or beliefs they may choose about these issues, but they are not admissible for the sake of public moral deliberation.[1]

Rather, we must create a bland or neutral public vocabulary, reflecting what John Rawls describes as an "overlapping consensus" on a set of minimalist and largely unspoken values. Because a pluralistic society is comprised of various communities holding contending visions of the common good, political and social stability requires "reasonable" public structures or procedures that deflect and neutralize potential conflict. In short, the common good can be effectively promoted only by refusing to endorse or privilege any single vision of the good. As Rawls admits, this commitment to public moral neutrality "removes from the political agenda the most divisive issues," but it is the price that must be paid to maintain a peaceful and well-ordered society.[2] With respect to stem cell research, for instance, we may disagree over the moral status of the embryo but agree that such research will result in the development of highly beneficial therapies. Consequently, our task is to hammer out policies regulating this research that we can, through the give and take of compromise, both live with while avoiding any distracting discussion of our disparate views on the moral status of embryos.

Although I acknowledge that there are short-tern advantages in this approach for addressing policy questions in an expeditious manner, the costs are too great in terms of long-term consequences. Over time, the so-called public square becomes increasingly vacuous as increasingly complex issues are reduced to the lowest possible common denominator among an increasingly diverse range of private interests. Indeed, the very nature of public moral deliberation becomes transformed from assessing the veracity of competing claims and arguments to concocting the best strategy for silencing one's opponents while marshaling support from as wide a coalition of interests as possible. Or, to paraphrase Alasdair MacIntyre, it is waging civil war with words (or better, slogans and sound bites) rather than weapons.[3]

What is lost in this scenario is the possibility that the process of public moral debate itself might lead to discovering something previously unknown or overlooked that might alter, broaden, or deepen our understanding of our life together as a public or the life of those communities and associations that comprise and embody our public life. Nor is the possibility entertained that through public deliberation we might actually encounter a truth that would require us to refrain from doing certain things despite the clamoring of public opinion. Instead, public moral deliberation becomes a tactical exercise of silencing or outmaneuvering the opposition, or, in George Grant's apt phrase, public controversy takes the "form of a struggle for political power rather than a debate between members of a common society."[4]

In practical terms, for example, I do not believe that most individuals and interest groups entering the public debate over embryonic stem cell research do so with an assumption that they might be persuaded to change their minds or that they will change the opinions of their opponents. Rather, they enter the fray in search of a strategy that will most effectively mute their opponents' claims, while simultaneously appealing to those who are at present undecided. Under these circumstances, the best role a religious community can play is to offer spiritual aid and comfort to those partisans attempting to shape public opinion that best approximates its own particular beliefs and convictions.

One may object that my admittedly uncharitable characterization of the current state of public moral discourse is not as bleak as I portray it. Although a pluralistic society necessitates a relatively thin or minimalist understanding of public life, we are compensated by potentially rich moral lives of private families, communities, and associations. The cold sterility of intermittent interactions with "strangers" (which are by nature procedural) does not diminish the moral solidarity and deep sense of meaning shared with "friends."[5] Nor does the procedural character of public moral deliberation necessarily eviscerate the quality of the normative commitments and values that we share with like-minded people. Individuals troubled by the prospect of creating and destroying embryos for the purpose of research, for example, are free not to use the resulting diagnostic or therapeutic treatments that are developed. And in turn they may find a comforting solace, or even a sense of moral superiority, in a community sharing similar misgivings and ideals that reinforce their refusal to benefit from an "immoral" medical practice. We can, after all, have a naked public square that is nonetheless filled by individuals richly adorned by widely varying attire.

This reassuring objection is misleading on two accounts. First, it assumes that the quality of public life, however thinly it might be conceived, is somehow unrelated to the normative convictions of the "private" associations and religious communities comprising civil society. The objection fails to recognize that the vitality of public life is directly proportional to the strengths of these associations and communities, and to insist that they strip themselves of their core convictions in their interactions with "strangers" is ultimately to diminish the life of the public they are seeking to form or maintain. The price of admission to the realm of public moral discourse is that the rich fabric of normative vocabularies formed by particular traditions must be shed in favor of an ethical Esperanto. Following Jean Bethke Elshtain, this requires a presumption that public moral discourse based on highly abstract procedural considerations is somehow "real," whereas the moral life of private associations and communities of daily encounters with actual people is somehow "unreal" in comparison. Yet this process ignores, if not reverses, the very nature of moral formation, for how we come to think about and value an embryo is largely formed in our relationships with concrete people rather than through abstract concepts, but these convictions have no currency within the "reality" of the public arena.[6] Thus, it is not surprising that moral debate in an increasingly vacuous public square is apparently conducted more by ghostly apparitions than by flesh and blood human beings.

Second, and more tellingly, the alleged neutrality of public moral discourse is largely illusory. To spare ourselves the "tyranny of principles" in the current debate over stem cell research, the practical consideration at stake is allegedly to determine what we may and may not lawfully do with a human embryo. It must be noted (and noted well) that we are being asked to ponder the fate of embryos *in isolation* from any procreative, parental, and familial contexts that have traditionally been the settings from which they derive their moral significance. Presumably thinking about an embryo as a glob of cells in a petri dish provides the kind of neutrality that will better enable a practical consensus over its eventual fate and proper use. Abstracting an embryo out from these social and moral contexts, however, is not a neutral act but a political stratagem, reflecting what Grant describes as a pervasive technical rationality that perceives the human good in terms of asserting its mastery over nature.[7] For how the public debate over stem cell research has been conducted to date is not so much over embryos per se, but rather embryos in light of our technological potential to exploit them for the sake of more beneficial medical treatments. The practical consideration at stake is how to perceive and portray a human embryo in a manner that will allow this promising research to be conducted without offending the moral sensibilities of too many tender souls. Thus, the fixation on issues such as setting a fourteen-day limit for conducting research or using only spare embryos that will be discarded anyway because they provide procedural distractions from the more pressing and inherently divisive question of the embryo's normative status.

Moreover, such a distracting and truncated public debate may very well have a corrosive influence on the vitality of so-called private moral life of those associations and communities we were assured could thrive along the edges of the neutral public square. For if members of a religious community, for instance, want to influence legislation or policy formulation governing embryonic stem cell research, will they not be tempted to reformulate their normative claims about embryos in terms that lend themselves more easily to manipulating trends of public opinion rather than reflecting a depth of conviction? And is it not the case that succumbing to such temptation is ultimately an injustice, because we do not take those outside our communities with enough seriousness to honestly share, or even confront them with, what we believe is good, and right, and true? Is the stratagem of distracting and thereby ultimately silencing the neighbor really very different than simply disregarding the neighbor?

An Alternative Approach to Public Moral Debate

What might the kind of public moral debate envisioned in this essay look like in terms of embryonic stem cell research? Answering this question would require a detailed analysis of contending religious convictions and moral claims, as well as a highly imaginative interpretation of how various interlocutors might contend with each other more as members of a common society than political partisans—a task that is far beyond the scope of this chapter, as well as the patience of the reader. Yet we can perhaps catch a glimpse of the type of conversation envisioned by reflecting momentarily on how the basic positions in this debate have already been staked out.

Proponents were quick to enumerate the medical benefits and miracle cures that would be developed for treating a wide range of debilitating illnesses and injuries. To emphasize the urgency for this research, a number of affected celebrities made highly visible appeals for federal funding as their last hope for restored health. Moreover, we were almost constantly reminded that the embryos that would be used for this research were microscopic, little larger than a pencil tip, thereby implying that nothing of any real significance would be destroyed. The contrast was striking: tiny specks of cells versus healing men and women who had become a part of our lives through movie and television screens. Opponents of embryonic stem cell research are not only crude Luddites, but also cruelly indifferent to the suffering of their fellow human beings.

Opponents were equally quick to remind us that all of us start our lives as embryos. Although this research might revolutionize health care, it did not justify the wanton destruction of human beings at their earliest and most vulnerable stage of development. Consequently, this research was tantamount to murdering unborn children, and we were treated to the spectacle of toddlers being displayed on television while a voice asked which one should have been killed for the sake of medical research. The contrast was again dramatic: are we willing to kill in order to save the lives of others? Proponents of embryonic stem cell research are not only arrogantly placing their faith in medical science, but are callous predators preying on unborn children.

Unfortunately, most of the official statements formulated by various churches and religious organizations to date have fallen into this pattern of rhetorical positioning. On the one hand, the United Church of Christ's (UCC) resolution in support of federally funded research on embryonic stem cells (see appendix E) recounts recent developments in genetic research and its promising medical applications for treating a wide spectrum of debilitating and life-threatening illnesses. Moreover, it simply asserts that, because scientists insist that embryonic sources of stems cells are clearly superior to adult sources, all frozen embryos destined to be discarded should be used to advance this research. Consequently, opposing embryonic stem cell research would be tantamount to resisting a progressive effort to relieve the suffering of literally thousands of afflicted individuals.

On the other hand, the Southern Baptist resolution on human embryonic stem cell research (see appendix D) calls for a total ban on federally funded research on human embryos, decrying it as "crass" utilitarianism and violating basic principles of human rights. Moreover, in stark contrast to the UCC resolution, it asserts contrary scientific evidence that adult stem cells offer more promising research applications than do embryonic stem cells. What is disappointing about both of these representative resolutions is the virtual absence of any theological or religious rationale for their respective positions. Except for a vague reference to the healing ministry of Jesus in the UCC resolution and an equally vaporous allusion to human beings being created in the image and likeness of God in the Southern Baptist resolution, there is no indication whatsoever of how theological convictions or religious beliefs inform their respective positions. Rather, both resolutions position themselves in respect to policy outcomes they wish to endorse in the ensuing political debates but offer no religious or moral insight that might contribute toward a richer or deeper understanding of the various issues at stake. Thus, perhaps unwittingly, both resolutions reinforce the perception that religious perspectives are not admissible in the arena of public moral discourse and that the only language that really "counts" is inherently political and procedural.[8]

Although such rhetoric may be effective for drawing initial battle lines by capturing headlines and thirty-second spots on the evening news, it does little to promote anything resembling genuine moral dialogue and debate. Would not the public have been better served if both sides had displayed, early on, a little more modesty and a little less hyperbole? Proponents largely failed to mention that there is in fact no way of knowing in advance whether embryonic stem cell research can ever deliver the miracle cures promised, much less in time for those currently afflicted. And although opponents expressed a passionate commitment to protecting human beings at the most vulnerable stage of their existence, they appear unable to extend the same sentiment to those suffering incurable diseases and injuries. The most troubling aspect of the rhetoric employed by both camps, however, has been their misdirection over what is purportedly the principal object of their dispute, namely, that the human embryo is surely something more than a speck of cells but that it is also clearly something less than a child. It is precisely by entering this ambiguous stage of human life to deliberate on the moral status of the embryo that would transform the current exercise of political maneuvering into a public debate. For such a debate would force us *as a public* to deliberate and come to terms with the finitude, frailty, and vulnerability that characterizes human life from beginning to end, particularly in terms of the natural *and* social affinities that bind us together and enable us to perpetuate civil society over time.[9] Yet if the goal is to win a political battle rather than inspire conversation, such a tactic is foolhardy, for too much ground is conceded too early in the contest.

Is there any compelling reason to believe that if religious communities take my advice they could change the moral course and tone of the public debate over embryonic stem cell research that we are now entering? Is there any hope of transforming it from a political war into a conversation over the common good? I have partaken too deeply of the theological and philosophical schools of realism to be overly optimistic, but I believe it is nonetheless worth the effort. It is my hope that it will be recorded that, in the debate over embryonic stem cell research, at least some religious communities chose to argue from the strength of their convictions rather than employing stratagems for swaying public opinion and, furthermore, that they adopted this approach not to trump the opposition but to promote a dialogue resulting in a richer fabric of public moral discourse, a dialogue requiring attentive listening, as well as taking the risk of having one's convictions changed, transformed, and possibly even enriched in the process.

Such an alternative is needed especially in the case of embryonic stem cell research, for if embryos come to be popularly perceived, at least partially, as biological commodities, the already fragile bonds that bind us together as a public (particularly in regard to its weakest and most vulnerable members) will be further strained. Or, in more prosaic terms, the most appropriate contribution that religious communities can offer in this debate is to insist that we not rush too quickly to plunder embryos for their health care benefits, and playing this important role requires the strength of conviction rather than an effective political strategy.

Acknowledgments

I am indebted to Steve Long, Andy Watts, and Tripp York, for their comments and criticisms of an earlier draft of this essay.

Notes

1. See Albert R. Jonsen and Stephen Toulmin, *The Abuse of Casuistry: A History of Moral Reasoning* (Berkeley: University of California Press, 1988), 1–20.

2. See John Rawls, *Political Liberalism* (New York: Columbia University Press, 1996), 133–72.

3. See Alasdair MacIntyre, *After Virtue: A Study in Moral Theory* (Notre Dame, Ind.: University of Notre Dame Press, 1984). Cf. Oliver O'Donovan, *The Desire of the Nations: Rediscovering the Roots of Political Theology* (Cambridge: Cambridge University Press, 1996), 283.

4. George Grant, *Technology and Empire: Perspectives on North America* (Toronto: House of Anansi, 1969), 46.

5. For analysis of the differing moralities of strangers and friends, see H. Tristram Engelhardt, Jr., *The Foundations of Bioethics* (New York: Oxford University Press, 1996), 74–81.

6. See Jean Bethke Elshtain, *Public Man, Private Woman: Women in Social and Political Thought* (Princeton, N.J.: Princeton University Press, 1981).

7. See Grant, 11–34.

8. In respect to the quality of religious statements, two notable exceptions include the statement of the Pontifical Academy (see appendix A) and the Theologian's Brief (see appendix G).

9. For a discussion of these affinities in respect to social and political ordering, see O'Donovan, 262–68.

THREE

The Ethics of Human Stem Cell Research

GENE OUTKA

Hype tempts us all. It would be naïve to exempt scientists from sometimes overstating the promise of their research. Early claims about what
gene therapy would accomplish, for example, arguably were exaggerated and
eroded public confidence. Yet claims about what stem cell research may accomplish belong in a class by themselves. The general public is now convinced that something momentous is occurring.[1] Both professional and popular publications register the excitement scientists evidence. This research, it
is routinely said, not only will expand significantly what we know about cellular life, but also will bring dazzling clinical benefits. Those who suffer from
Alzheimer's disease, Parkinson's disease, and the like are regularly identified
as eventual beneficiaries. The cumulative effect is to raise expectations generally to a high pitch.

Whether these claims will prove exaggerated awaits research efforts that
have only just begun.[2] As a society, we long for such benefits and sense a genuinely other-regarding motive among those who make these claims. That
is, the prospect that such research will bring concrete benefits to numerous
human sufferers motivates scientists to engage in it. At the same time, we recognize that less altruistic consideration—e.g., a search for windfall financial
profits—sometimes operate as well.

Yet, concern about profits figures only marginally in the ethical controversies that this research has generated so far. Rather, the controversies show

how a single other-regarding motive that accents benefits to human sufferers cannot and should not go unexamined. Even as we praise the motive, we confront a host of complicating questions. May research that accents benefits to human sufferers trump all other considerations as it seeks to secure these benefits? What of embryos and aborted fetuses? Should their value reduce *totally* to their importance for relieving the suffering of *third* parties? Can a readiness to do anything with and to embryos and aborted fetuses be acceptably other-regarding after all? What other moral considerations count, and how much should they count?

I approach these questions by assuming a diagnosis of ourselves as human beings that sets the terms for appraising even novel developments. Two basic generalizations about us that derive from this diagnosis influence my reflections in what follows.

First, we are *morally capable* creatures, *accountable* beings. We should assume responsibility for what we are doing, and we go wrong when we seek to deny our agency. Not every outcome in stem cell research is foregone; we may shape, as well as be shaped by, developments, and much may depend on initiatives we take that accord with our own convictions. Second, we are creatures who can *exalt ourselves inordinately*—i.e., in ways that flout God and manipulate others. This condition is called *sin* and *moral evil* in many religious communities. Reinhold Niebuhr takes sin to extend in two directions:

> The Bible defines sin in both religious and moral terms. The religious dimension of sin is [our] rebellion against God, and [our] effort to usurp the place of God. The moral and social dimension of sin is injustice. The ego which falsely makes itself the center of existence in its pride and will-to-power inevitably subordinates other life to its will and thus does injustice to other life.

To be tempted to usurp and to do injustice is endemic to human life as we know it. In my own identity as an Augustinian Christian, I take it that we are continually in danger and that everything is corruptible.[4] If this is right, one should expect that stem cell research is itself not immune to pressures that may usurp and do injustice. In short, stem cell research presents novel opportunities and challenges and manifests permanent capabilities and dangers.

In examining the ethical controversies that surround stem cell research, I canvass a spectrum of value judgments on sources, complicity, adult stem cells, and public and private contexts and explore how debates about abortion and stem cell research converge and diverge. I propose extending the principle of "nothing is lost" to current debates, and I locate a definitive normative region to inhabit, within a larger range to rival value judgments. The creation of embryos for research purposes only should be resisted, yet research on "excess" embryos is permissible.

Recurring Ethical Controversies

Four points assume special salience in discussing the collision of value judgments pertaining to stem cell research. Three points concern the "sources" of stem cells. Particular evaluations of the three tend to cohere internally. That is, how disputants evaluate the "status" of the embryo and aborted fetus (point one) relates to how they evaluate "complicity" (point two) and "the alternative of research on adult stem cells" (point three). Comparison of a spectrum of particular evaluations increases understanding of where disagreements lie.

The fourth point concerns the political and legal contexts in which this research proceeds, and specifically proposals about how such research should be organized, financed, and overseen. They do not receive the rigorous examination that characterizes debates about "sources," but their importance is obvious. They impel us to mesh what is ethically desirable with what is politically viable. I can only touch on such an immense subject in this paper. But to ignore institutional realities altogether, including institutional lacunae, amounts to a certain kind of ethical failure, one that holds at bay questions about which institutional arrangements conduce to the "common good."

Moral Judgments Pertaining to the Sources of Stem Cells

In this section, I review a spectrum of moral positions that pertain to the *status* of the fetus and of the embryo; the question of *complicity*, where research depends on *someone* destroying a fetus or an embryo; and the *alternative* of concentrating on stem cells found in *adults*.

Views on the "Right"

Here I refer mostly to Richard Doerflinger, who defends in lucid prose Vatican instruction on human procreation. Yet, other communities, including many evangelical Protestants and (Eastern) Orthodox Christians, hold these views as well.[5]

The status of fetuses and embryos. Doerflinger considers the moral status of the human embryo in light of the historic conviction that each human individual has basic and equal human worth. No differences in talents or other conditions should overturn this evaluation. If one takes this evaluation to heart, one infers that no one should be treated, exhaustively and without remainder, as a means or instrument. "The human individual, called into existence by God and made in the divine image and likeness, . . . must always be treated as an end in himself or herself, not merely as a means to other ends. . . ."[6] It is cogent to infer inviolability, too. To kill the innocent deliberately and directly is *the* prime instance of going against such inviolability. Fetuses and embryos are assuredly innocent. Doerflinger sees both abortion and the destruction of embryos merely as means to other ends and as going against inviolability.

By maintaining that the moral status of fetuses and embryos is decisively similar, he combats a view that certain liberal Catholics (among others) espouse, in which "conception" differs from "individuation." In this view, the early embryo is relevantly formless until the "primitive streak" appears at about 14 days of gestation. Proponents argue that one otherwise cannot account for the possibilities of "twinning" and "fusion" that occur after conception.[7] Consequently, this view allows moral room for maneuver up to 14 days. Doerflinger replies that the most recent studies show that the early embryo is not simply formless, that the capacity for twinning is established very early indeed, and, in any event, that the overwhelming majority of embryos lack the property of spontaneously producing twins. A more general concern surfaces as well. Some hold that, *even* if the argument from "twinning" allows for nontherapeutic experimentation, it remains the case that stem cell research regards early life only as "manipulable stuff"—not as a child, but as an entity that merely serves other, albeit perhaps laudable, ends. Such attention, it is argued, jeopardizes the ability to welcome children into the world and to care for them.[8]

Complicity. Doerflinger reviews and assesses various arguments about complicity in the act of harvesting stem cells. Here certain differences between abortion and the destruction of embryos *do* appear, but they give no comfort to the advocates of research on embryos.

Doerflinger considers efforts that Congress has made since 1993 to distinguish the actions and intentions of those who abort fetuses from the actions and intentions of federally funded researchers who use the resulting fetal tissue in human transplantation.[9] Although he does not altogether approve of these efforts, or of some of the arguments urged on their behalf, he grants that a researcher who uses fetal tissue does not necessarily support the decisions to request or to perform an abortion.

He refuses to say the same, however, about the derivation and use of stem cells from embryos.

> Here those who harvest and use the cells are necessarily complicit in the destruction of the embryo. This is illustrated by the fact that, if embryonic stem cell research were governed by the same legal conditions that now govern the use of fetal tissue from abortions in federally funded research—e.g., harvesting to be done only after death, researchers' needs may not determine the timing and manner of the destruction of the fetus—the research could not be done at all. These stem cells are taken from embryos while they are still living. In effect, the harvesting of cells is itself the abortion—i.e., it is the act that directly destroys a live embryo—and the method of destruction, using microsurgery to extract the embryo's inner cells from the outer trophoblast, is determined entirely by the needs of the stem cell researcher.[10]

Given this assessment, he rejects as incoherent any claim that government funding of research on embryonic stem cells does not involve complicity in the destruction of embryos as long as researchers did not participate directly in such destruction. This distinction strikes him as little more than a "bookkeeping exercise," since the act of destruction is not only *presumed* as with research on aborted fetuses, but is directly *undertaken* as part of the research protocol.

He also criticizes the argument that derivation of stem cells from "spare" embryos donated by fertility clinics differs morally from using embryos created *solely* for research purposes and that only the latter uses embryos as a mere *means* to other peoples' ends. Doerflinger maintains that destruction of an entity for body parts because that entity will die in any case is not the same as using cells from an entity that is already dead. In addition, "a policy that permits research only on 'spare' embryos is virtually impossible to maintain in practice. Fertility clinics easily can produce a few more embryos from each couple, ostensibly for reproductive purposes, to ensure that there will be 'spares' for research at the end of the process"[11]

The alternative of adult stem cells. Doerflinger accents the advances that researchers have made in the work on adult stem cells. One major advantage of using adult cells on which everyone agrees is the avoidance of possible tissue rejection by treating a patient with his or her own cells. That researchers cannot say with certainty that research on embryonic cells will yield clinical applications that would not be available otherwise strengthens the case on practical grounds for limiting research attention to adult stem cells. We as a society thereby avoid putting *firmly*, and probably *irrevocably*, into place morally contestable practices that may not be clinically necessary.

Views in the "Middle"

The status of fetuses and embryos. A more liberal case is made within the Catholic tradition that favors human embryo stem cell research. It requires one to distinguish, as I mentioned earlier, between conception and individuation. Margaret Farley[12] accepts this distinction. For her and a number of other Catholic moral theologians, the human embryo is not considered in its earliest stages (prior to the development of the primitive streak or to implantation) to constitute an individualized human entity with the settled inherent potential to become a human person. The moral status of the embryo is, therefore (in this view), not that of a person, and its use for certain kinds of research can be justified. (Because it is, however, a form of human life, it is due some respect—for example, it should not be bought or sold.)[13] While accepting some embryo research, she commends certain safeguards—e.g., donors may not specify who is to receive stem cells for therapeutic treatment, and an "absolute barrier" should be maintained between therapeutic and reproductive cloning.

Complicity. Those who occupy positions in the middle may disagree about the moral standing of fetuses, but they tend to agree on the moral relevance of one distinction respecting embryos. They refuse to equate the destruction of embryos who already exist, but who will either be frozen in perpetuity or discarded, with the creation of embryos solely for the purpose of destroying them in an effort to benefit third parties. Complicity in the former instance looks morally less ominous. For the decisive role here is played by those responsible for the existence of embryos and for the decision to freeze or discard them. Researchers react rather than initiate, after those responsible have reached their fateful determinations. Some estimate that at least 100,000 frozen spare embryos in the United States alone now languish in *in vitro* fertilization clinics. The majority are no longer wanted or claimed. They will never be implanted. Judging complicity should reckon with this datum.

The alternative of adult stem cells. Those who occupy middle places along the spectrum are disposed generally to accept—though sometimes reluctantly— a verdict that many scientists have reached. Stem cells derived from adults are necessary but not sufficient—if one wants to maximize the data available and hence the possibility of breakthroughs—to support all clinically important areas of research. Research using each of the "sources" should go forward, for each has its own advantages and disadvantages, and they complement one another. The settled verdict is that embryonic stem cell research holds promise for which at the present there is no adequate substitute.

Views on the "Left"

Here I refer mostly to the work of John Robertson.

The status of fetuses and embryos. Those who stand on the left side of the spectrum characteristically deny that the value accorded to previable fetuses should *ever* override pregnant women's choices to terminate their pregnancies for whatever reason. To attribute basic and equal human worth to each human individual requires more than the presence of cells that have the potential to develop into a person. Robertson extends this value judgment to embryos in the following way:

> [Those] holding this view about pre-viable fetuses view preimplantation embryos, which are much less developed than fetuses, as too rudimentary in structure or development to have moral status or interests in their own right. . . . No moral duties are owed to embryos by virtue of their present status and . . . they are not harmed by research or destruction when no transfer to the uterus is planned.[14]

Robertson refuses to say, however, that because embryos lack moral status in their own right one may do anything *at all* with them. They are not "means" in this sense or to this extent—e.g., one may not use them "for toxicology testing of cosmetics" or buy and sell them. One can deny intrinsic value to all embryos and still accord them "symbolic" value and "'special respect' because of their potential, when placed in a uterus, to become fetuses and eventually to be born."[15] Nevertheless, this symbolic value should be trumped when necessary to pursue a good scientific or medical end that cannot be pursued by other means.

Complicity. Robertson thinks that any distinction between the derivation and the use of embryonic stem cells does not survive critical scrutiny. Researchers who use stem cells derived from embryos are complicit in their destruction, regardless of whether they participate directly in the act of destruction. Moreover, those who support the use of cells from spare embryos from *in vitro* fertilization clinics should *also* support the creation of embryos for the purpose of research. In both cases, embryos *do* become a means to address the needs of others, once one decides to use them in research. In this regard, Robertson displays an ironic affinity with Doerflinger. Both insist on an either/or scenario, though of course each draws the opposite normative conclusion. *Either* one should stop opposing the creation and destruction of embryos for research purposes only (in Robertson's view), *or* one should oppose not only the creation and destruction of embryos for research purposes, but also the research on spare embryos from *in vitro* fertilization clinics (in Doerflinger's view). Pressures are exerted on those in the "middle" from the "left" as well as from the "right."

The alternative of adult stem cells. Those who take the position Robertson does can prefer limiting research to adult stem cells only *if* such a limit in fact will yield superior therapeutic benefits overall. The criteria for making this determination are, it seems, empirical and consequentialist: what research on which sources will produce the greatest benefit overall? Given this, Robertson insists that at present no definitive empirical-consequentialist case exists for limiting research to adult stem cells. The most promising course is to pursue research using cells from each of the three "sources"—fetuses, embryos, and adults.

Ethical Considerations in Political and Legal Contexts

I now turn to the fourth realm in which ethical controversies recur, the political and legal realm. Two areas of controversy figure most prominently here. The first concerns controversies about federal funding of stem cell research. These consume the bulk of disputants' energies to date. Passions rise highest where taxpayer dollars figure centrally. Disputants perceive federal expenditures to attest to society-wide convictions. Those who occupy particular positions along the spectrum characterized in the foregoing sections battle on behalf of criteria for federal funding that support their respective normative conclusions about "sources." A pastiche results.

The second area concerns controversies about the absence of coordination between research permitted in the public and private sectors. I find it worrisome that research possibilities lack any sort of society-wide oversight. Yet many either welcome the status quo or appear resigned to it. Some judge the current arrangements to be desirable on the whole, at least they prefer to leave well enough alone, so long as researchers are free *somewhere* to pursue various research possibilities. To enjoy liberty from scrutiny allows those in the private sector to conduct research that might achieve major breakthrough, but which societal scrutiny might forestall. Others judge the present situation to be ad hoc to a fault. They accept that publicly and privately funded research should be coordinated somehow. Nevertheless, they view the practical chances of coordination to be distressingly slight.

Normative Assessments

In this section, I evaluate more fully the positions described so far, which requires that I also indicate positions I am myself disposed to take.

I commend as a normative point of departure the conviction that Doerflinger[16] cites: "the human individual, called into existence by God and made in the divine image and likeness, . . . must always be treated as an end in himself or herself, not merely as a means to other ends." Many hold this conviction, not only those on the "right." To regard each person for his or her own sake, as one who is irreducibly valuable, authorizes a sphere of inviolability, as previously noted. It also heightens sensitivity to multiple ways one may go wrong—e.g., when one dominates, manipulates, and self-aggrandizes. To affirm inviolability and to abjure domination captures deeply important commitments. They direct moral attention along lines I take to be permanently valid.

Many likewise draw on the language of ends and means to evaluate cases of "killing and saving."[17] To commit murder is arguably the quintessential instance of going wrong. Those who murder arrogate to themselves a position of false superiority. They usurp or perversely imitate God, who alone is the "Author of life and death." Yet they possess the power to accomplish this. That is, in the case of murder, they *can* do what they *ought not* to do. They also effectively claim that they are better than their victims, so much better that they are prepared to "instrumentalize" them through and through. Murderers do their victims *incommensurable* harm; in depriving them of life, they reduce them to "mere means" to their own aims and projects. Those who save life do the opposite. They pay homage to what they take the character of God's love to be, by attesting that the one saved is not a mere means, but someone for whom they should care, whose well-being they should protect and promote.

To mix theological and Kantian ingredients in this way deserves a degree of examination that I cannot pursue here.[18] I focus now on how far this evaluation extends. Is it cogent to claim that abortion and embryonic stem cell research are morally indistinguishable from murder?

Posing so blunt a question concentrates our thoughts, but it also encourages an unfortunate tendency to restrict evaluative possibilities to a single either/or. Either one judges abortion and the destruction of embryos to be *transparent* instances of treating fetuses and embryos as mere means to others' ends or one judges abortion and embryonic stem cell research to be, *in themselves*, morally *indifferent* actions that should be evaluated *solely* in terms of the benefits they bring to others. I reject such a simplifying restriction. The most fitting place to inhabit is, I think, a *particular* region in the "middle." Here one engages the formidable arguments from both the "right" and the "left" and appropriates as much as one consistently can, but still retains a distinctive vantage point. From this point, one finds a position *less* cogent than many conservatives do that extends *simpliciter* (morally, if not legally) the prohibition of murder to the prohibition of abortion and embryonic stem cell research. But one ascribes *greater* importance to fetuses and embryos than many liberals do, an importance not reduced to the benefits that research on them may bring to third parties. I shall say more about this region as the most fitting place to be, while acknowledging the dangers in locating oneself there.

From the "Right": Specificity and Stringency

The tradition of moral reflection that shapes conclusions on the "right" emphasizes two considerations, specificity and stringency, that those in the "middle" should heed as well.

Specificity. I am drawn to the strand in the tradition that endeavors to identify certain actions—which persistently affect our weal and woe—in a definite and nontautological way. To consider the action that concerns us most: murder is prohibited, but not all killing is murder. How should one discriminate? One should not do so by writing morally evaluative references into the characterization of what murder is, for then one renders this characterization morally decisive by definition. So, for example, murder is defined as "wrongful" or "unjust" or "irresponsible" killing. But resorting to tautology forecloses debate. The tradition favors instead specification that leaves the wrongfulness of the action open, to be "settled only by a further nondefinitional judgment."[19] The prohibition of killing in the Decalogue is construed more precisely to mean that one should *not intentionally kill innocent human life*. This construal specifies what "murder" is. It is a delimited action-kind. The judgment that murder in *this* sense is wrong purports to be true, yet is not a tautology. (I accept that who is requisitely "innocent" is sometimes difficult to ascertain and deeply controversial, but not in the cases before us here.) It is the judgment under scrutiny, and it remains possible to dispute it.

To construe more precisely the prohibition of killing introduces, on the one hand, a certain flexibility. It helps to make sense of society's organized efforts to provide security for its citizens against arbitrary, unprovoked, or otherwise unjust assaults on life and limb and to accommodate policing, courts of law, and soldiering. We should by no means idealize here; activities that fall under these organized efforts are always corruptible, and, in some measure, distinctively so. Recognition of corruptibility, however, need not undermine the efforts. Yet, on the other hand, this construal limits flexibility. When one meets cases that fall within its range of applicability, one may not go roaming around redescribing at will. Instead, one acknowledges the moral features of the case at hand and either condemns the action or seeks special justification or mitigation.

Stringency. To reiterate an ancient question: May we (ever) do evil to achieve good?[20] Cases that fall within the prohibitions range of applicability present one with two choices: the prohibition against killing as precisely construed possesses either *absolute* or *prima facie* authority in any circumstance to which it applies.

A familiar historical example brings out the difference between the two kinds of authority. President Truman reasoned that to drop atomic bombs on Hiroshima and Nagasaki would serve to hasten the end of the war and cost fewer lives than a full-scale invasion of Japan.[21] We cannot ascertain whether he was empirically correct, but we can ask whether he was morally right that the criterion of "fewer lives lost" should trump. Those who adhere to the prohibition against killing as precisely construed normally extend it in circumstances of war to forbid the direct and intentional killing of noncombatants (as "material innocents"). To accord *absolute* authority to the prohibition thus extended means that Truman erred morally when he calculated total outcomes in the fashion he did. No argument from outcomes—which includes Truman's readiness to pursue a "countercity" rather than "counterforce" strategy to shorten the war and to kill fewer persons—can override what by prior determination is judged to be wrong in itself to do, whoever does it. In this sense, one may never do evil to achieve good. To accord prima facie authority to the prohibition thus extended means that noncombatant immunity has presumptive validity. This is strong enough to query Truman's decision. There is a presumption in the prohibition's favor, and any violation has the burden of proof. The prohibition retains authority in that it may never be disregarded in a circumstance to which it applies, but only overridden, and always with compunction. Still, one may consider in tragic cases whether one should do something morally repellent—something one would not do for its own sake—to prevent something far worse.

Unless one understands how the prohibition against killing is construed, and that it may be accorded absolute authority, one fails to grasp where and why many on the "right" judge abortion and embryonic stem cell research as they do, and where and why many on the "left" demur.

Those on the "right" judge that the prohibition extends to fetuses and embryos. Both are *innocent*, and aborting a fetus and disaggregating an embryo are *direct* actions that kill. Whether death is strictly *intended* is a more complicated question in the case of abortion. Certain defenders of abortion claim that a pregnant woman may justly withdraw her bodily life support from the fetus, but that she may not thereby have a "right" to the fetus' death, if the fetus can survive outside her womb.[22] Before 20 weeks of the pregnancy, however, this distinction has strictly theoretical interest. Death accompanies withdrawal of bodily life support, whatever hypothetical speculations one appends. Death also accompanies the disaggregation of embryos, which affords no room for distinguishing between intending withdrawal but not death. As for "human life," the last part of the specified prohibition, those on the "right" maintain that each human entity, from the time of conception, is irreducibly valuable. Indeed, each is judged to have an equally protectible status. If embryos are currently genderless and removed from the naked eye, they differ from the rest of us only in that they await implantation, growth, and subsequent entry into the world of social interaction.[23] They contain the requisite genetic information that renders each unique, and *all* of us began at this stage. Why then discriminate? Does self-absorption blind us to injustices we may commit because at present we enjoy superior power? Assuredly, fetuses and embryos cannot fight back on their own behalf, but *none* of us could at the point of our origins. We transcend self-absorption when we revere human entities by doing nothing that would jeopardize their inviolable status, just as our parents earlier revered ours and fought for our survival when necessary. To intervene and destroy fetuses and embryos palpably intrumentalizes them for the sake of those who are presently stronger. We would do well to remember what our parents did, and that we are grateful for what they did, when we evaluate abortion and embryonic stem cell research.

Those on the "right" move from specificity to stringency. One should make others' ends one's own, *provided that these ends are morally permissible.* Violating the prohibition against killing as precisely construed *is* an impermissible end. One may not do or approve *this* evil, even when it achieves good. For one should always relate any benefits one aims to secure to what one is prepared to do to obtain them. One does best to consider *first* what *one does* and forbears, and not simply what will *happen*, and to live within the absolute limits that the prohibition against murder sets for us.

In the "Middle": Potentiality and When "Nothing Is Lost"

I have identified arguments from the "right" that I find formidable, yet I also find certain extensions of them less cogent than their defenders assume. Two lines of argument prevent my concurring that abortion and embryonic stem cell research are morally indistinguishable from murder and permit my occupying a particular region in the "middle."

Potentiality. The first line of argument concerns "potentiality," as applied to fetuses and embryos. This word recurs in the literature, yet is a red flag to many on the "right" and on the "left." Conservatives think it nullifies a serious commitment to fetuses and embryos; liberals deride it as "mere" potentiality, a referent too indeterminate ever to be permitted to trump decisions to abort and to conduct research on embryos. The truth, it seems to me, is complicated in ways these contrary evaluations neglect.

I claim that "potentiality" is double-sided in a way that leads me to draw back from unqualified extensions of moral status, but to draw back a lesser distance than do those on the "left." It yields appraisals that show how debates about abortion and about embryonic stem cell research are sometimes allied and sometimes not. How they diverge especially needs to be recognized. I consider these claims in turn, and attend first to fetuses.

One side of "potentiality" registers what fetuses *are not yet*, at least during the first 20 weeks of the fetus' existence (or until the lungs are sufficiently developed). The fetus *cannot* live absent total physical dependence on one and only one person in all the world. Assuming the medical technology available now and in the foreseeable future, pregnancy involves unique physical dependence. Every pregnant woman is noninterchangeable. *No one and nothing else can take her place.* This state of affairs is not at all odd (not numerically uncommon), yet it is distinctive (though numerically common). The distinctiveness means that in certain respects pregnancy is *sui generis.* Analogies that are entirely satisfactory do not exist.

Consider two sorts of cases in which this total dependence leads on to ascribe to the fetus a status less than that of equally protectible human life when weighed against the pregnant women, who also is *an end in herself.*

The first sort of case involves parity-conflicts in which one physical life collides with another, and it is impossible to save both. Such cases include conflicts between the pregnant woman and her fetus, where the pregnant woman will die unless the life of the fetus is terminated (though thankfully such cases are now rare). A random lottery solution lacks advocates in this set of circumstances. In brief, such a case differs from lifeboat scenarios, because, unlike the latter, one does not propose drawing straws. Rather, one unhesitatingly saves the pregnant woman. "Potentiality," here, captures the sense that commitment to fetal life is prima facie, not absolute. One may override the commitment when the fetus imperils the pregnant women's physical life. Parity-conflicts of this sort are resolved in one way.

The second sort of case involves encounters with evil, where a woman is pregnant as a result of rape or incest. Here the absence of satisfactory analogies asserts itself most forcefully. No one except the pregnant woman can carry in her body someone conceived in rape, but nontransferable just the same, who combines her own genes with those of her violator. She is uniquely near the fetus, yet is alienated from it by virtue of the crime, which affects her intimately and in which she is not complicit. This evil case brings three factors together. The first concerns unique dependency. The woman can help in a way no one else can. The second concerns agency. She is not responsible for being pregnant. The third concerns cost. She carries the offspring of violence. The first holds for all pregnancies. The second and third do not, and they go together. How far these three factors are severally necessary as well as jointly sufficient to set this case apart points to the intricacies of debates about abortion as such that I cannot address here.[24] But at least in this case, to judge that a woman is obliged to bring the fetus to term exceeds what the conditions of her own inviolability accommodate. Potentiality again stops short of equal protectibility that would prohibit termination in every such instance.

The second side of "potentiality" registers what fetuses *are*. Here I take potentiality to be something more than mere possibility. The "more" refers to an entity actually in motion, a force that is there, a *power underway* (after the primitive streak and implantation). This power includes *existent* capacities to *acquire* in the future various characteristics typically attributed to those who "bear the human countenance"—e.g., self-awareness, personal accountability, and conscious relations with other human beings. Since fetuses possess the capacities to acquire these characteristics, traditional appraisals are correct that fetuses have a value greater than zero, a value separate and independent from their parents.[25] In short, they *are* irreducibly valuable. I take this to mean that, from conception forward, a presumption holds that they should come to term. Overriding this presumption carries the burden of proof.

Such commitment to fetal life makes theological sense to many for whom biblical passages count in weighing matters of life and death. Believers adduce passages that trace the working of providence back to the womb (see, for example, Isa. 44:2; Ps. 138:13, for Jews and Christians; Luke 1:31–39, 42–44, for Christians). One should not dismiss citations like these as mere "proof-texting." For they cohere with a conviction that God's covenant love stands as our alpha and omega. In this case, human love should correspond to far-reaching providential action. To err on the side of inclusiveness looks fitting. That a biblical depiction of providence encompasses potentiality implies that human love should start before recipients become self-aware.

These evaluations of the status of the fetus locate me on the right side of the tortured "middle," within the vast territory of debates about abortion. It is essential to make these evaluations explicit, if one hopes to add anything useful to the widely-voiced opinion that debates about stem cell research chiefly reprise debates about abortion. This opinion is right in that both fetuses and embryos *are* irreducibly valuable—i.e., both have a value greater than zero, a value separate and independent from their parents; and still neither can live and develop without total physical dependence for a period of time on one and only one person in all the world.

Yet the opinion misses divergences that I find important in staking out a particular region in the "middle" of the smaller but rapidly expanding territory of debates about stem cell research. I allude to three such divergences here. The first concerns the kinds of *conflict* at issue. The second concerns the parameters of *cost*. The third concerns the range of *choices* that present themselves. I discuss each in turn.

First, debates about embryos *in vitro* miss the characteristic tensions resident in the two sorts of cases just reviewed, where total dependence allows one to ascribe to the fetus a status that is less than equally protectible human life when weighed directly *against* the pregnant woman. For these cases focus on conflicts between two parties where a one-to-one correspondence obtains. While the stakes differ—saving one physical life by ending another and deciding whether a fetus conceived in rape should be brought to term and parented with all of the deep and permanent commitments this carries— the correspondence does not. It is otherwise with *in vitro* embryos. In typical circumstances, no similar conflicts exist. Although one takes an active step by transferring the embryo, an act that the two conflict cases do not require and a stage that they have, in any event, passed beyond, the decision to transfer is not a conflicted one. The circumstances here center on infertile couples who want a child and who embrace emphatically the deep and permanent commitments parenting brings. If a conflict emerges, it is neither immediate nor one-to-one between the fetus and the woman. Rather, it is between those embryos who are not transferred and are to be frozen in per-petuity or discarded and the needs of *third* parties who suffer from various maladies that research on embryos *may* eventually alleviate.

Second, the costs (harms) are the same for fetuses and for embryos but diverge notably in the case of pregnant women and third parties suffering from maladies mentioned earlier. Fetuses aborted and embryos disaggregated both undergo *incommensurable* physical harm—i.e., lethal harm beyond human powers to reverse or compensate. I argue elsewhere that this incommensu-rable harm constitutes a decisive similarity between abortion and infanticide, and one may extend this argument to embryos.[26] As already discussed, con-servatives judge this similarity to fall under the prohibition against murder and accord the prohibition absolute priority. I do not go so far. At the same time, one should not shrink from soberly acknowledging the similarity itself. By contrast, important divergences surface when considering costs to preg-nant women and third parties suffering from maladies. Recall the instance of pregnancy following rape. The woman is not *obliged* to carry a fetus con-ceived in these circumstances to term. Yet she may choose to do so out of extreme generosity and despite excruciating personal cost. The sacrifices she makes are hers, though after the fact. That is, the rapist deprives her of the exercise of her agency, and yet she exercises it *post eventum;* she may choose voluntarily to bear the cost. This sort of personally incurred cost disappears in case of third parties suffering from maladies that stem cell research may al-leviate. I do not deny that they suffer excruciatingly as well and that allevi-ating their suffering is something to be lauded. Still, their standing as possi-ble beneficiaries of embryonic stem cell research is unrelated to the circumstances of conception. They are not actors within *these* circumstances. Unlike a pregnant woman, they cannot connect the plight they face with what they *do*, at voluntary cost to *themselves*. Moreover, no researcher on stem cells currently suffers, or faces permanent changes to his or her future life, that compare at all with the suffering a woman knows whose pregnancy is due to rape, and who elects to bear and parent a child.

Third, the choices a woman confronts whose pregnancy is the result of rape are stark. Either she elects to terminate the pregnancy or she does not, and, if she does not, she bears the child and may either place the child for adoption or parent. Her reasons for deciding as she does may vary, from hon-oring her own inviolability to honoring the well-being of the fetus who is another innocent. Yet some one reason must trump these others. And the time to decide is short: if she does not terminate, she will bear, by affirma-tion or default. Whatever she decides, she will live with a host of physical and emotional affects, from a single point of origin. Once more, the circumstances surrounding stem cell research diverge markedly from her case. The reasons to conduct such research include the alleviation of suffering and the advancement of scientific knowledge. Neither reason must trump; they may reinforce each other. And the choices of how to pursue such research are several, as the debates about stem cell "sources" make clear. No one source is the narrow gate through which all promising lines of research *must* pass. One can debate the relative advantages and disadvantages of each, as well as the place of moral constraints. Finally, the decision is not forced by a fixed timeline. And these are early days of such research.

The respects in which debates in which debates about abortion and about stem cell research converge and diverge push those in the "middle" in contrary directions, as already observed. Some are disposed to be *more* permissive about embryonic stem cell research than about abortion for these reasons: (1) Prior to implantation one may distinguish conception from individuation; and (2) after implantation the fetus is indeed a "power underway," who, left to self-elaborating processes, is likely to become "one of us." Abortion actively intervenes to terminate "a force that is there" and has the burden of proof, whereas an embryo *in vitro* must still be transferred, and, until it is, one cannot describe it *now* as a self-elaborating power underway.

Others are disposed to be *less* permissive about embryonic stem cell research than about abortion, for this reason: abortion may involve bona fide direct conflicts between two entities who *are* both ends in themselves, whereas embryonic stem cell research is *morally* simpler. It concerns only one entity about whom one can say with certainty, here and now, that the action one takes, disaggregation, causes incommensurable harm. That third parties may benefit from the research subsequently done is an outcome for which one fervently hopes, but such benefit lies in the future. And we cannot gainsay the possibility that it may be attained without taking any lethal step—e.g., though research on other, morally unambiguous, sources of stem cells (from adults, umbilical cord blood, and the like). The doubled-sidedness of potentiality supports the less permissive side, it seems, yet one should weigh a further argument that furnishes some room for maneuver and nuances the distinctiveness of debates about embryonic stem cell research.

"Nothing Is Lost"

A second line of argument prevents my saying that abortion and embryonic stem cell research are morally indistinguishable from murder and permits me to occupy the particular region in the "middle" I do: "nothing is lost."

Here I invoke and extend the "nothing is lost" principle. I first learned of this principle from Paul Ramsey. While he was committed to an absolute prohibition against murder as the intentional killing of innocent life, he was prepared to attach two *exempting conditions* to it. One *may* directly kill when (1) the innocent will die in any case and (2) other innocent life will be saved.[27] These two conditions stipulate what "nothing is lost" means. They originally extend to parity-conflicts, where one physical life collides directly and immediately with another physical life, and one cannot save both. (Ramsey may not have continued to uphold the principle in later writings, and I doubt in any case that he would have accepted the further extension I now offer.) I will argue, however, that it is correct to view embryos in reproductive clinics who are bound either to be discarded or frozen in perpetuity as innocent lives who will die in any case and those third parties with maladies such as Alzheimer's and Parkinson's as other innocent life who may be saved by virtue of research on such embryos.

I grant this extension *at best* stretches the "nothing is lost" principle nearly to the breaking point. For I defend the extension (and perhaps the original principle) as a move to the effect that (1) nothing *more* is lost, and (2) *less* is lost, or, at least, *someone* is saved. This extension is worth considering because stem cell research represents a particular instance of a general phenomenon, namely, that novel developments arise for which no clear moral precedents suffice to guide us. In such cases, one should seek both to extend traditional moral commitments and to incorporate new developments as cogently as possible. To labor the obvious: some of the controversies have arisen only *after* the age of *in vitro* fertilization dawned. *It* stands behind them, amplifying questions about "ends" and "means" that our forebears could not foresee. Unless one is prepared now to repudiate *in vitro* fertilization as such, so that one sympathizes with infertile couples but refuses them a *right* to overcome their condition by any means that science and their financial resources make available, one must take the moral measure of these new possibilities.

In the instance before us, I sympathize with the plight of infertility, but I am disquieted by the way *in vitro* fertilization is practiced in our culture. I will return to this disquiet. But, rightly or wrongly, "excess" embryos are a tenacious datum, for they are a result of the practice as it currently exists in the United States. I welcome the day when such necessity vanishes and welcome in the meantime "adopting" mothers willing to implant embryos, when the genetic couple consents.[28] Not to welcome these events belies the claim that embryos as well as fetuses are irreducibly valuable. Nevertheless, it looks at present as if embryos in appreciable numbers will continue to be discarded or frozen in perpetuity. *They will die, unimplanted, in any case.* (Nothing *more* will be lost by their becoming subjects of research.) Again, it is the absence of prospects for *these* innocents that partly extends the first exempting condition. It is the enhancement of prospects for *other* innocent life that partly extends the second exempting condition. (*Less* will be lost, or, at least, *someone* may benefit.) These judgments taken together summarize the case I wish to make.

I say "partly" extends, not "wholly" and certainly not "transparently." The case for extension I put forward shows both continuities and discontinuities with prior judgments on the ethics of direct killing. I take the prior judgments seriously and extend them to novel situations as far as I can. But I also acknowledge that the present debates on embryonic stem cell research involve a moral space that is, to a degree, unprecedented. I shall give two examples of the continuities and discontinuities I have in mind.

First, a point of continuity: My extension goes so far, and no further. It includes embryos conceived to enhance fertility, but who will never be implanted. It excludes embryos created exclusively for research, where one intentionally creates them for the sake of benefits to third parties that one hopes to secure and where one *embraces* the disaggregation of embryos as necessarily part of what *one does*. This limited extension accords with the "timbre" of "nothing is lost" in that one encounters circumstances that one did not initiate and that one wishes were otherwise. That one contemplates doing repellent things, things that one would not do for their own sake, indicates how intentional killing was not "part of the plan" from the start. This timbre matters, yet a difference presents itself even here. The parity-conflict cases assume a contingent disaster that no one intends or foresees, nor that is part of any established procedure. The circumstance of *in vitro* fertilization includes a recognition that "excess" embryos are, to date, endemic to the procedure in the United States. At a minimum, this is foreseen. Still, the intention of the procedure is to alleviate infertility, not to create embryos for research. Thus, a significant continuity holds, despite this difference.

Second, a point of discontinuity: The "nothing is lost" principle, as originally formulated, is narrower and more exact than an extension of it to the novel case of unimplanted embryos can be. In the sort of parity-conflict cases that goaded those in the past to articulate the "nothing is lost" principle in the first place, unless one directly kills one of the parties, one cannot save the other. This allows for the claim that one *would* save both if one *could*. No similar temporal and causal limits apply to the case of unimplanted embryos. No other party will directly and immediately die if one elects to save embryos by freezing them. Any "conflict," as previously stated, is much further removed and comparatively indeterminate, plainly from parity-conflict cases, and arguably from abortion decisions more generally.

From the "Left": Derivation and Use and Ends and Means

Although the particular location in the "middle" that I seek to inhabit has led me so far to pursue boundary questions on the "right" side, what I have said anticipates how I shall pursue boundary questions on the "left" side as well. I noted previously that Doerflinger and Robertson, as representatives of each side, sometimes concur that the moral choices are less complicated than I take them to be. They hold respectively that *either* one should oppose not only the creation and destruction of embryos solely for research purposes, but also the employment of spare embryos in research, *or* one should stop opposing the creation and destruction of embryos for research purposes only. I have sought to show morally relevant differences between the creation and destruction of embryos for research purposes and the use of spare embryos in research. To the degree these differences make sense, they suggest how those in the "middle" differ from those on the "left" as well as from those on the "right." I now examine these boundary questions more closely.

Derivation and Use

Robertson makes two claims, noted previously in the discussion of "complicity," that should not be conflated. He contends first that the distinction between derivation and use is chimerical. Researchers are complicit in destroying embryos when they use stem cells derived from them, regardless of whether they personally engage in the act of destruction. So far, I agree. The NIH guidelines promulgated during the Clinton administration split the difference, perhaps for legal reasons and to promote civil peace by not ignoring conservatives' concerns altogether, while funding research all the same.[29] Second, Robertson contends that, if one supports research on "spare" embryos, one should support the creation and destruction of embryos solely for the purpose of research. For embryos do become "mere means" once one decides to use them in research. I think one may compatibly accept Robertson's first contention and reject his second. And if I am right to extend, in a qualified way, the "nothing is lost" principle, one has important reasons to reject the second.

To recount the reasons clarifies where boundaries lie. Such reasons focus on what status one ascribes to embryos and on how one interprets the injunction to treat persons as ends in themselves.

Ends and Means

Regarding status, recall that Robertson holds, along with many others, that embryos are too rudimentary to have moral status in their own right. He ascribes "symbolic" value to them, which means, for example, that they may not be bought and sold, but they lack "intrinsic" value. By contrast, the account of potentiality and irreducible value that I have offered does ascribe status to them in their own right. This account warrants resistance to such a thin view of their value that virtually any reason—except qualms about commercialization—trumps it. I intend potentiality to be robust enough, in the case of both fetuses and embryos, to resist the view that fetal life and embryonic life lack any weight that might ever be determinative *as soon as* their value conflicts with other values. Without such resistance, concern for such life is reduced to a platitude, a mere expression of goodwill, that never has efficacy, that can always be trumped.

Regarding the injunction to treat persons as ends in themselves, Robertson insists that, once we decide to use embryos in research, they do become a "mere means." This announces moral equivalence between two circumstances that I have argued differ relevantly. It is one thing to say that innocent life "will die" in any case, when one refers to a condition that one did not, by one's own hands, bring about and that in most instances one cannot alter. It is another thing to say that innocent life will die at one's own hands, a condition that one plans and brings about from the beginning and where one could have done otherwise. This latter procedure does reduce embryos to a menial status through and through. One would distort the "nothing is lost" principle beyond recognition if one proposed to "extend" it to say that nothing is lost when one creates an entity whose prospects are nil because of what one intends from the start.

The difference is there, yet Robertson's insistence valuably presses one to ask: How much remains of the injunction to treat persons as ends in themselves when one allows research on frozen and eventually-to-be-discarded embryos? I reply that the normative force of the injunction diminishes significantly when one takes to heart *their* prospects. It diminishes for everyone, not only for those who allow research. Some seek to witness to the dignity of embryos by refusing to do anything to them other than to freeze them. They adhere to the norm I mentioned when canvassing conservative views, that one does best to consider *first* what one does and forbears, and not simply what will *happen*. Although this norm counts for me across a range of other circumstances, I find in the present circumstance that such a witness threatens to idle in relation to what the injunction paradigmatically summons us to undertake. It is difficult to specify what interest one *protects and promotes*, for example, when freezing and discarding are all that one can seriously envisage. To honor potentiality, where there is no hope of implantation, is to honor *perpetual potentiality*.[30] It diminishes *action-guiding content*, either present or future, in the injunction to treat as an end. It even affects what is said in the theological context to which I alluded earlier concerning providence and corresponding love. For one cannot precisely equate the affirmation that love should start before recipients become self-aware with an affirmation that one should love recipients who will *never* become self-aware. To deny equation is emphatically not to disbelieve in providence in both cases, and it is not to withhold corresponding love in both cases. It aims only to acknowledge that the room for exercising fidelity in action over time may differ. What one can and cannot do in treating persons as ends will be affected by *their* prospects. Love for an embryo who will live at most in a perpetually frozen state without self-awareness has less prospective room than love for a fetus who is a power underway and who eventually *will* acquire self-awareness. What one can envisage and do, now and later, has a greater scope in the latter instance, which is why termination obliterates a future that the fetus now *has* in prospect, a future that an embryo frozen in perpetuity *lacks*.

This severely diminished force bears on the second exempting condition, that other innocent life will be saved. The case to extend this condition is imperfect as well, indeed more so, for reasons already given. I observe, however, that as one disallows the intentional creation of embryos for research purposes, one draws more closely together the moral considerations weighted in judging the permissibility of research on fetal cadavers and certain-to-be-discarded embryos. In both cases, the genetic parents decide whether to donate them for research. Researchers play a lesser role—they lack a voice in the decision to abort or to attempt *in vitro* fertilization—than when *they* guide the intentional creation and destruction of embryos.

Political and Legal Contexts

I ask next how the normative orientation of locating oneself in the "middle" affects one's engagement in the political and legal contexts in which stem cell research proceeds. Four broad observations must do for the present.

Range of applicability. First, the range of applicability of such an orientation needs to be clarified. Do I take it to be relevant to the entire body politic, at least in the United States, or only to certain segments of it? I divide this question into two parts.

(1) Since I referred to Augustinian Christian convictions at the start, do I address persons in the church only, or persons in the wider society also? The answer is that, in this instance, I address neither audience exclusively. On the one side, particular convictions influence how I depict the orientation in various ways. For example, I have in view certain Christian accounts of agape-love as I interpret the notion of persons as ends in themselves;[31] I extend a principle from Ramsey, a Christian writer who claimed that his own formulation of "nothing is lost" came from a Christian understanding of charity; I dwell on the prohibition against murder as precisely construed; and my senses of "intentional" and "innocent" are influenced by my own tradition. On the other side, the subject of stem cell research demonstrably engages the wider society, and much of the literature on moral issues and scientific developments that I have read and incorporated focuses on no religious tradition. Moreover, to cite examples again, the prohibition against murder is one on which Jews, Muslims, and secularists likewise have innumerable things to say, from which I have learned; the protection of citizens from murder is a basic duty of *any* political government, which partly explains the urgency of debates about whether abortion and/or embryonic stem cell research are morally indistinguishable from murder; and the maladies that may be cured or ameliorated through stem cell research fall within the range of common human woes—e.g., Alzheimer's disease may strike anyone, regardless of whether one is a religious believer.

(2) Does the orientation apply with equivalent normative force in the public and the private sectors? It does, "in principle," but insofar as "ought implies can," the prospects in American society for de facto adherence differ greatly. I alluded to some of the reasons much earlier. Disputants from all parts of the spectrum have concentrated chiefly on what federally funded research should include. Comparatively little has been said about research conduct in the private sector. Some liberals especially look now to the private sector for much of the most promising and innovative research. As they see it, for the government to issue and enforce rules that would apply to *all* research would be a poison gift. To implement such a step would curtail substantially the kinds of research presently allowed in the private sector. They prefer to rely instead on ethical standards propounded by the professional bodies most directly involved and on the type of ethics advisory committees that Geron and

the Advanced Cell Technology group, for instance, have established. These matters are beyond the scope of the present enquiry. I add only that one need not attack indiscriminately all free market undertakings in this area to entertain certain justified worries. The results of privately funded research may not be immediately or universally available to the general public in the fashion that federally funded research is. In addition, "commercial organizations" are, of course, designed to make money. Neither in their objectives nor in their management are they designed to balance conflicting interests or to pay homage to the distinctive noncommercial qualities of medical research and medical care. The government, at a minimum, should not ignore the paucity of coordination I mentioned previously or permit so many decisions to be made by default.

Ongoing moral debates. Second, the subject of stem cell research remains volatile. It so far resists any repetition of the pattern that one sometimes sees, where theorizing about moral matters yields divergent and rival points of departure and lines of argument, but weighing political possibilities and institutional policies yields more agreements and points of consensus (a modus vivendi of sorts). One should beware of assuming here that, once one turns to institutional policies, there is no longer a need to engage in "theoretical" debates. One's moral point of departure determines, in key part, what one takes desirable and undesirable institutional policies to be. One makes claims, as I have done here, weighing arguments about where to place oneself along a spectrum and exploring how far judgments about abortion and stem cell research diverge, and so on. If one gives these enduring moral concerns short shrift, one enters the political fray with undefended assumptions that one merely announces.

To avoid such an outcome, one must not grow weary of moral debates. They matter, and views taken exert vast influence. Between those who evaluate embryos as equally protectible human life and those who evaluate embryos as only "clumps of cells in petri dishes," there is no peace. I have tried to suggest why neither of these evaluations is adequate, and I must continue to attempt to address conservative and liberal objections to my position. For example, conservatives may discern a consequentialist flavor in the "nothing is lost" principle (the innocent *will* die in any event; other innocent life *will be* saved). I claim it is fitting to ask, in the case at hand, what *actual* benefits are or might be conferred and on whom. Yet I hardly comment on the intricacies of consequentialist theories. I only consider actual benefits in the case presented by the anomalous practice of *in vitro* fertilization, which results in entities whose destruction was not directly intended from the start. Liberals may protest my refusal to keep concern about the status of embryos in circuit with every other morally estimable consideration, without benefit of even prima facie ranking. While I extol possible benefits to third parties from embryonic stem cell research, I resist allowing concern about the status of embryos to recede again to a platitude, where it never has efficacy and can always be trumped.

Overall orientation. Third, I should specify further the overall orientation that emerges from the particular location in the "middle" that I inhabit. To extend the "nothing is lost" principle in the way I do sets a deontological constraint on "sources" that applies in principle to stem cell research in the public and private sectors. It draws a line between research on embryos created solely for this purpose and research on embryos from *in vitro* fertilization clinics that are to be discarded or frozen in perpetuity. It disallows the first sort of research and allows the second. This constraint makes concern about embryos more than an ineffectual afterthought. One should acknowledge any costs it may incur. Some liberals worry for instance that such a limit might affect adversely the "quality" of available embryos for research, a difficulty that intentional creation for research would surmount. Researchers debate whether this worry is well-founded empirically, but if one is unwilling to risk this much, one again transmutes concern about the status of embryos into a mere expression of goodwill. If one holds the constraint hostage to interminable bargaining, one deprives it of a normative force that makes a discernible difference. The line should remain intact, and one should be content to derive as many scientific and medical benefits as possible from research on "excess" embryos.

The constraint matters as it marks the drawing of a line. It matters also as it registers an attitude of ongoing mourning for a plight. One thus regards research, even on excess embryos, as something to which one only reluctantly acquiesces. This attitude begins in sympathy for those who view their own infertility as an affliction they seek to overcome. It continues in allowing unprecedented *in vitro* technology that sometimes triumphs over this affliction, but such technology brings with it one foreseeable and lamentable outcome, namely, the presence of embryos to be discarded or frozen in perpetuity. One welcomes neither infertility nor excess embryos. The attitude concludes in a desire that one day there will no longer be a need to destroy embryos. That is, one looks forward to a time when it is possible to reprogram adult stem cells so that embryos are no longer required as a source. One further hopes that this time comes quickly, that the establishment of cell lines will make the use of donated embryos a transitional matter. In short, to destroy embryos *never* should leave one at ease or become simply unproblematic, a permanently acceptable part of routine procedures. Our society's research priorities should attest to such an attitude.

A "performative" danger. Fourth, when I claimed initially that the most fitting place to inhabit is a particular region in the "middle," I said there were dangers associated with that position. Let me give one example of such a danger.

This example falls within my third broad observation, that the constraint draws a line and registers an attitude. The danger derives from practical undermining more than from outright repudiation. Here the overused metaphor of "slippery slope" comes into play. One recalls Doerflinger's contention that researchers and those in charge of *in vitro* fertilization clinics might in effect collude to produce by the "back door" spare embryos in accordance with research needs rather than an intention to alleviate infertility. The "slope" at issue is not so much one of theoretical argument, where the "logic" of a position one takes moves inexorably to conclusions one deplores. It is more "performative." That is, the line—between research on embryos created solely for this purpose and research on embryos slated to be discarded or frozen in perpetuity—is accepted provisionally by some on the "left," perhaps because fewer public qualms presently accompany concentration on spare embryos, but their passion lies in the benefits to third parties this research promises. To participate in collusion, therefore, occasions no crisis of conscience on their part. Their governing aim is to secure embryos for research. If the line one day evaporates, they will have little to lament. In the meantime, their task is to exploit the distinction as far as possible, to make the most of all the opportunities for research it can possibly yield. The pressure to go down this slope shows how a line is harder to maintain when the attitude of permanent unease toward research on embryos is not shared.

Concluding Remarks on "Nothing Is Lost"

I said at the beginning that two basic generalizations about human beings inform my reflections in these pages. We are morally capable creatures, accountable beings, and we are creatures who can exalt ourselves inordinately, in ways that usurp and do injustice. The debates about stem cell research that I have canvassed and evaluated attest to the relevance of both generalizations in one particular space where, as I also said, one meets novel opportunities and challenges, as well as permanent capabilities and dangers.

Yet the results of canvassing and evaluation here display varying grades of moral clarity and accountability and different kinds of usurpation and injustice. I conclude by summarizing and elaborating such results in one concrete instance, my attempt to apply the "nothing is lost" principle to debates about stem cell research.

I proposed to apply the principle against a background of claims about *the status of human life from conception forward.* I take conception and all that it alone makes possible as *the* point at which one should ascribe a judgment of irreducible value. Once conceived, each entity is a form of primordial human life, a being in its own right, that should exert a claim upon others to be regarded as an end rather than merely means *only.* One should view its potentiality as constituting a presumption in favor of its coming to term. If this presumption is not robust enough to trump other claims on at least some occasions, the judgment of irreducible value becomes a platitude. "Symbolic respect" stands too near the chimerical because it trumps little or nothing *whenever* conflicts occur.[32]

After conception, I find no comparable bright line, but defend some proximate discriminations. Before individuation and implantation, the entity does not yet have the full-fledged moral standing of a fetus. Yet, for its part, a fetus' value is not equally protectible with the pregnant woman's, for she too is an end in herself and has developed beyond the potentiality that still characterizes the fetus. Equal protectibility holds after the fetus becomes capable of independent existence outside the womb.

These claims about status indicate why I deny that abortion and embryonic stem cell research are morally indistinguishable from murder and why I deny that abortion and embryonic stem cell research are morally indifferent actions in themselves, to be evaluated wholly by the benefits they bring to others.

The claims indicated as well why I object to the sort of embryonic stem cell research that creates embryos for the sake of benefits to third parties, where one *embraces* the disaggregation of embryos as *necessarily* part of what *one does.* To conduct such research clashes directly with the judgment that entities conceived have irreducible value. It is one thing to accept that one need not ascribe full moral standing or equal protectiblity to embryos. It is another thing to "instrumentalize" them completely through actions that are performed solely for the potential benefit of *third* parties. But the claims also indicate why I object to the ironic alliance that those on the "right" and "left" sometimes form, to the effect that one either should forbid all embryonic stem cell research or permit it all. There is, I believe, a more nuanced possibility, where one may distinguish *creating* for research from *employing* for research. The latter allows consideration of the tangled aftermath of *in vitro* fertilization as a practice in our culture. Employment for research connects with the datum of discarded embryos, where the original creation of those embryos possesses a noninstrumental rationale, namely, the promotion of fertility. In this case, what one intends does not exhaustively concern benefits to third parties, yet the aftermath allows one to pursue benefits to third parties without embracing the disaggregation of embryos *from the start* as necessarily part of what one does. These differences lead me to argue that the "nothing is lost" principle illumines a morally significant distinction between creation for research and employment for research.

I offer four concluding observations that illustrate varying grades of moral clarity and accountability and different kinds of usurpation and injustice.

First, an appeal to "nothing is lost" remains distinct from the kind of calculus President Truman favored. He elected to take certain innocent lives intentionally for the sake of saving many more. If this kind of calculus operates in stem cell debates, as it surely does in certain circles, it should not be run together with "nothing is lost." The latter principle limits itself to two sorts of cases, neither of which possesses the type of balancing of lives lost and saved that Truman's calculus encompassed. In the first sort of case, one *can* choose whom to save, but one *cannot* save all. This sort of "life-boat" scenario requires the invocation of some distributive criterion—e.g., a lottery. In the second sort of case, one *cannot* choose whom to save. The embryos in question fall under the second case. They will be *lost* no matter what one does. They will die if one does nothing—one may assume that the embryos will be frozen and eventually destroyed, or at least that they cannot be kept in limbo forever—and one cannot save them by killing others or letting others die.[33]

Second, consider another reasonably clear but less widely recognized distinction regarding the status of moral claims. I believe my appeal to "nothing is lost" reaches a moral judgment that should endure rather than one that holds only "for the time being." It is one thing to seek both to extend traditional moral commitments and to incorporate new insights as cogently as possible in the development of enduring moral judgments regarding novel moral issues. It is another thing to seek the most judicious judgment deemed acceptable at the present time, where the judgment remains provisional and revisable in response to shifting social consensus. In the latter case, disputants sometimes tacitly assume and hope that what is beyond the pale now may not be later. I follow the former route. Once one takes the step of combining traditional commitments and incorporating new developments, one should reach definite moral judgments. If the principle that "nothing is lost" rules out the creation of embryos for research, but permits research on spare embryos, shifts in public opinion should not cause a change in course.

Third, consider a possible difficulty internal to the "nothing is lost" principle itself. Here clarity is harder to attain. The difficulty is that "nothing is lost" may permit more extensions than I seek. Recall the difference Doerflinger cites, which I noted much earlier: destruction of an entity for body parts because that entity will die in any case is not the same as using cells from an entity already dead. Some may worry that the principle may allow the general "harvesting" of organs or tissues from the living who are, for example, terminally ill, permanently comatose, or condemned to die by authorities of the state as criminals. The specter of Nazi doctors may well appear: If certain people are slated for death anyway, why not experiment on them to the point of ending their lives to acquire knowledge?[34] These possible extensions differ from the one I propose because the embryos in question are in physical limbo without history or prospects. I judge that the general difference Doerflinger cites should *otherwise* continue to claim allegiance. It *is impermissible* to destroy *any* entity for body parts who has an agential history even if he or she does not now have any considerable future—e.g., entities whose maturity—their "potentiality" has *long since* been realized—deprives their genetic parents of authority to end their existence or to elect to donate them for research. But the "perpetual potentiality" of the embryos in question distinguishes them markedly enough from these other entities. "Perpetual potentiality," assuming the claims I made about the double-sidedness of potentiality, permits one intelligibly to find more affinities than differences between fetal cadavers and the embryos in question. Whatever other extensions "nothing is lost" may warrant—e.g., in cases of tragic forced choices, which I have not considered at any length—the extension I offer here pertains to a peculiar case by virtue of what the embryos in question currently are and are not. John Reeder[35] observes in quoting Baruch Brody that "the basic point of nothing is lost is that, as Brody puts it, the one to be killed does not 'suffer any significant losses . . . in unrealized potential.'"[36] I claim that "unrealized potential" carries for the embryos in question *distinctive* finality that resists generalization.[37]

Fourth, another difficulty for "nothing is lost" derives from the very features that render this case peculiar. I ask now whether these features may complicate my proposed extension beyond what I have so far allowed. I only touched on what complicates when I registered "disquiet" over the way in which *in vitro* fertilization is practiced in our culture. It is the practice itself that gives possible trouble for my proposed extension.

The original conflict, as I noted earlier, is that one welcomes neither infertility nor excess embryos. Those who are spared infertility should show "epistemic humility" toward those not spared and should try to understand from a respectful distance their sense of deprivation. One thus rejoices in what is hardly a trivial gain: *in vitro* fertilization has overcome a condition that would have otherwise consigned many to having no genetic children of their own. One should remember this and feel the force of the conflict that has ensued.

Yet excess embryos remain a tenacious datum, too, and it is here that the disquiet centers. It persists on three levels. The first I noted when I contended that one should never regard as simply unproblematic the destruction of embryos or the consignment of them to perpetual storage. Furthermore, one should extend this attitude of permanent unease to research on them as well. Something inestimably valuable is at stake and at risk. A second level pertains to current practices in American society. Approximately 10,000 embryos are added each year in procedures and processes that are substantially free of society-wide oversight—a general circumstance I lamented previously—and in which the profit motive plays a large but ill-considered role. Although many embryos will be transferred, it is certain that many more embryos are generated than will be transferred. A third level concerns the moral diagnosis that accompanies these practices. Such practices are a human achievement, not a contingent natural disaster. Matters could have been otherwise.[38]

It would be idle to deny that such disquiet complicates my proposed extension. At a minimum, the permanent unease that I defend should not end in passive resignation to these status quo practices. Such unease should prompt instead far more critical and skeptical appraisals of the practices presently in place. Again, in this area the government is permitting too many decisions to be made by default.

Yet I continue to uphold my extension of "nothing is lost," albeit in a chastened mood, rather than jettison any distinction between the creation and the employment of embryos, as those on the "right" and "left" propose. My reasons are also three.

Above all, one should not avoid the brute fact of the 100,000 embryos or more who are languishing in vats and whose prospects for implantation are nil (and many are unviable). Even if *in vitro* fertilization stopped the creation of excess embryos immediately, this phenomenon confronts us. Accounts of "nothing is lost" allow for circumstances in which the fact that innocents will die is seen as a moral evil and not a natural accident—e.g., situations a tyrant creates. The reasoning is this. One need not approve of how the situation was created in order to judge that it is better to save some than none when those who die would die anyway. I regard employment of discarded embryos for research as morally tolerable, and no more. It remains difficult for me to see what treating them as ends summons us to do, how flushing them respects them more, or is less evil, than employing them for research.

Second, I grant that recognition of human construction of the *in vitro* fertilization industry puts pressure on my earlier distinction between a condition we did not, by our own hands, bring about, and in most instances cannot alter, and a condition where we plan and bring about the death of an innocent life at our hands when we could have done otherwise. Yet I draw back from any grand use of the societal "we" in this prior account of human construction. We, as individuals, may now become complicit if we do not criticize, yet the circumstances of the original construction attest to the realities of our social pluralism. Those most deeply affected—the infertile—and those prepared to respond—the organizers of the industry—were the driving forces behind such construction. So it continues to matter whether one creates these particular embryos and embraces their disaggregation from the start as necessarily part of what is done, or whether one only knowingly foresees that excess embryos form part of the practice.

Third, the particular region of the "middle" that I extol averts the excesses of a debate that engages those on the "right" and the "left" concerning the *necessity* of embryonic stem cell research. The former denies such necessity—there are alternative ways, even if slower ones—e.g., research on adult stem cells—that will bring the desired benefits—and the latter insists on it in order to alleviate immediate mass suffering as quickly as possible. I opt for something less sweeping. I bracket the debate about necessity. Instead, let us not elide the difference between creation and employment, but rather draw this line for good and permit research in accordance with it.[39]

The performative danger to which I have alluded will endure. Yet one may nevertheless defend certain commitments as always in force, such as the injunction to treat persons as ends in themselves. I think that the constraint I identified that follows from this injunction continues to do important normative work in calling attention to a limit and in lauding research within it. There is still lasting value in seeking moral integrity, after one engages—with critical respect—points on the spectrum.

Acknowledgments

Some of these pages began as the Wofford Lecture in Religion, Society, and Ethics, given at Wofford College in Spartanburg, South Carolina, on 26 September 2000. I am grateful to John Bullard, who issued the original invitation and kindly hosted me there. I thank Margaret Farley, Richard Fern, Wayne Meeks, Gilbert Meilaender, Paul Outka, John Reeder, Brian Sorrells, and Sondra Wheeler, for their reading of an earlier draft in its entirety. I also owe thanks to Ronald M. Green, who introduced me to important literature and with whom I had several stimulating conversations. Moreover, monthly meetings over a two-year period with the Yale Faculty Working Group on the Ethics of Stem Cell Research were indispensable. It was my good fortune to chair this group. We disagreed among ourselves on many occasions (sometimes vigorously, but never rancorously), and the others should not be held accountable for the views I articulate here. Still, my debts to these discussions are incalculable. The members for one or both years included John Booss, Robert Burt, Thomas Duffy, Margaret Farley, Arthur Galston, Myron Genel, Albert Jonsen, Robert J. Levine, Maurice J. Mahoney, Theodore Marmor, William F. May, Carol Pollard, Pasko Rakic, Dennis Specer, Michael Weber, and John L. Young. Finally, I received useful commentary and criticism from the President's Council on Bioethics, at its meeting on 25 April 2002, in Washington, D.C. I thank its members for the careful attention they gave to this paper, and its Chairman, Leon Kass, for inviting me and for advice I took on how to formulate one of my key claims more accurately.

Notes

1. For one early, engaging indication, see Gregg Easterbrook, "Medical Evolution: Will Homo Sapiens Become Obsolete?" *New Republic,* vol. 220, no. 9, 20–25.

2. Scientific uncertainties may go deeper than the public realizes. Maureen Condic (see "The Basics About Stem Cells," *First Things* 119 (January 2002): 30–39) asks whether the merit of embryonic stem cell research is as widely accepted by researchers as it is routinely alleged to be. She emphasizes the scientific and medical disadvantages of using embryonic stem cells and their derivatives in treating disease and injury and on the advantages of using adult stem cells, even though the latter field is not as far advanced. For a report that testifies to the volatility of current scientific judgments about the respective merits of adult stem cell and embryonic stem cell research, see Alex Dominguez, "Studies Cast Doubt on Efficacy of Stem Cells," *Nando Times* (13 March 2002) [available at http://nandotimes. com /healthscience/v-text/story/302144p-2637767c.html].

3. Reinhold Niebuhr, *The Nature and Destiny of Man, I* (New York: Charles Scribner's Sons, 1949), 179.

4. See Gene Outka, "Universal Love and Impartiality," in *The Love Commandments: Essays in Christian Ethics and Moral Philosophy,* edited by Edmund S. Santurri and William Werpehowski (Washington, D.C.: Georgetown University Press, 1992), 1–103.

5. See Gilbert Meilaender, "Remarks on Human Embryonic Stem-Cell Research," in *Ethical Issues in Human Stem Cell Research,* vol. 3, *Religious Perspectives* (Rockville, Md.: National Bioethics Advisory Committee, 1999), E1–E6, and Demetrios Demopulos, "An Eastern Orthodox View of Embryonic Stem Cell Research," in *Ethical Issues in Human Stem Cell Research,* vol. 3, *Religious Perspectives,* B1–B4.

6. Richard M. Doerflinger, "The Ethics of Funding Embryonic Stem Cell Research: A Catholic Viewpoint," *Kennedy Institute of Ethics Journal,* 9 (1999): 138.

7. This view holds that embryos up to 14 days are preindividual and prepersonal (see, e.g., Thomas A. Shannon, "Remaking Ourselves? The Ethics of Stem Cell Research," *Commonweal,* vol. 125, no. 21 [1998]: 2–3, and Richard A. McCormick, "Who or What is the Preembryo?" *Kennedy Institute of Ethics Journal,* 1 [1991]: 1–15). Shannon sees a distinction between cells drawn from a preimplantation embryo and cells drawn from an aborted fetus. I later compare stem cell research on embryos and fetal cadavers.

8. See William Werehowski, "Persons, Practices, and the Conception Argument," *Journal of Medicine and Philosophy* 22 (1997): 479–94.

9. See Doerflinger.

10. Ibid., 141.

11. Ibid., 143.

12. See Margaret Farley, "Roman Catholic Views on Research Involving Human Embryonic Stem Cells." In *Ethical Issues in Human Stem Cell Research.* Vol. 3, *Religious Perspectives,* D1–D5.

13. Ibid., D-4. Papers prepared for a meeting of the National Bioethics Advisory Commission (7 May 1999) display the diversity of views within religious traditions (National Bioethics Advisory Committee, 2000). (In addition to the papers already cited by Farley, Meilaender, and Demopulos, see Dorff, Pellegrino, Sachedina, Tendler, and Zoloth, in the same volume.)

14. See John A. Robertson, "Ethics and Policy in Embryonic Stem Cell Research," *Kennedy Institute of Ethics Journal,* 9, no. 2 (1999): 117–18.

15. Ibid., 118.

16. Doerflinger, 138.

17. See John P. Reeder, Jr., *Killing and Saving: Abortion, Hunger, and War* (University Park: Pennsylvania State University Press, 1996).

18. I try to sort out these ingredients elsewhere. (See Gene Outka "Respect for Persons," in *The Westminister Dictionary of Christian Ethics,* edited by James F. Childress and John Macquarrie [Philadelphia: Westminster Press, 1986], 541–45, and "Universal Love and Impartiality," in *The Love Commandments: Essays in Christian Ethics and Moral Philosophy,* edited by Edmund S. Santurri and William Werpehowski [Washington, D.C.: Georgetown University Press, 1992], 1–103.) To employ Kant's second formulation of the categorical

imperative here does not imply acceptance of Kant's moral theory as a whole. The formulation, as I treat it, distills Christian depictions of neighbor-love.

19. See John Finnis, *Moral Absolutes: Tradition, Revision, and Truth* (Washington, D.C.: Catholic University Press of America, 1991), 37.

20. See Richard A. McCormick and Paul Ramsey, eds., *Doing Evil to Achieve Good* (Chicago: Loyola University Press, 1978).

21. Moral assessments of Truman's decision are legion (see, e.g., G. E. M. Anscombe, "Mr. Truman's Degree," in *Ethics, Religion and Politics: The Collected Philosophical Papers of G. E. M. Anscombe,* volume 3, 62–71 [Minneapolis: University of Minnesota Press, 1981]; Michael Walzer, *Just and Unjust Wars* [New York: Basic Books, 1977], 263–68; Jonathan Glover, *Humanity: A Moral History of the Twentieth Century* [New Haven, Conn.: Yale University Press, 2000], 89–112; and, with reference to stem cell debates, Gilbert Meilaender "The Point of a Ban; Or, How to Think about Stem Cell Research," *Hastings Center Report,* vol. 31, no. 1 [2001]: 9–16).

22. See Judith Jarvis Thomson, "A Defense of Abortion," *Philosophy and Public Affairs,* 1 (1971): 47–66.

23. See Andrew Sullivan, "Only Human," *New Republic,* 30 July 2001, 8.

24. I gesture elsewhere to the intricacies of these debates (see Gene Outka, "The Ethics of Love and the Problem of Abortion." Second Annual James C. Spalding Memorial Lecture, printed in booklet form by the School of Religion, University of Iowa, Iowa City, 1999). Although I incorporate several sentences from this booklet in my present account of abortion, I simplify the issue by focusing on the case of rape; I do not consider here the moral responsibilities that arguably arise from requisitely voluntary sexual relations.

25. See John T. Noonan, Jr., "An Almost Absolute Value in History." In *The Morality of Abortion: Legal and Historical Perspectives,* edited by John T. Noonan, Jr., (Cambridge, Mass.: Harvard University Press, 1970), 1–59.

26. Outka, "The Ethics of Love and the Problem of Abortion."

27. See Paul Ramsey, *War and the Christian Conscience: How Shall Modern War Be Conducted Justly?* (Durham, N.C.: Duke University Press, 1961), 171–91.

28. It is important to qualify any generalization that the creation of spare embryos is endemic to *in vitro* fertilization procedures as such. Consider the case of Germany since the passage of the 1990 Embryo Protection Act (Embroynenschutzgesetz [EschG]); the text is available online at www.bmmmmgesundheit.de/rechts/genfpm/embryo/embryo.htm). Germany allows during an *in vitro* fertilization procedure only the number of embryos to be developed beyond the pronucleus stage that will later be transferred. And three is the maximum number of transfers permitted. The striking result is that Germany faces no "plight" of excess embryos. To be sure, there is a drawback. "Success rates" are lower than they are in the United States. Nevertheless, I conclude two things. First, the normative position I espouse in this chapter effectively pushes closer toward the policies that Germany follows. These would require, however, a degree of regulation that is needed but missing in the United States. Second, this same normative position requires that I attend to the large number of excess embryos that exist already in the United States and in certain other countries. Their "plight" is a fait accompli. The "nothing is lost" principle

that I invoke here pertains chiefly to their plight. To ignore the existence of these excess embryos, to fail to reflect on their significance, would subtly belittle the moral quandaries they pose. I am indebted to Sabine Hermission for information about policies in Germany. More generally, see also my last remark in the final section of this chapter.

29. These NIH guidelines have now been withdrawn. On 20 November 2001, the NIH posted the Human Embryonic Stem Cell Registry. It lists the human embryonic stem cell lines that satisfy the eligibility criteria specified by President Bush on 9 August 2001. These criteria are more restrictive than required by the position I defend here, for they "allow Federal funds to be used for research on existing human embryonic stem cell lines as long as prior to his announcement . . . the derivation process . . . had already been initiated" (see National Institutes of Health, NIH Human Embryonic Stem Cell Registry. [Bethesda, Md.: NIH, 2001]. Available at http://grants.nih.gov/grants/guide/notice-files/NOT-OD-02-005.html and at http://escr.nih.gov/.) This should be compared to the earlier comprehensive report and recommendations of the National Bioethics Advisory Committee.

30. Brian Sorrells suggested this phrase while reading an earlier draft, and I thank him for this as well as other suggestions that improved the paper significantly.

31. See Gene Outka, *Agape: An Ethical Analysis* (New Haven, Conn.: Yale University Press, 1972).

32. Those who endorse "symbolic respect" for embryos rarely ask directly whether this respect should ever trump when it conflicts with the welfare of third parties, except for repeating qualms about commercialization. Michael Meyer and Lawrence Nelson (see "Respecting What We Destroy: Reflections on Human Embryo Research," *Hastings Center Report, vol. 31, no. 1 [2001]: 16–23) offer a fuller discussion, however, as they defend* the claim that one may respect embryos even as one intentionally destroys them. One may, because the moral status of embryos is "weak or modest." Although they are "alive" and "valued, in some cases very highly, by many people," they are not "agents," or "persons"— prior, at least, to "individuation" around 14 days—and they lack "ecological significance" (18). Destruction should occasion, nevertheless, a sense of "regret and loss" (20). My judgments differ from theirs at two points. First, I claim that the irreducible value embryos have trumps the possible welfare of third parties in that one may not create embryos where one embraces their disaggregation from the start as necessarily part of what one does, for this instrumentalizes them through and through. Meyer and Nelson (21) stress that as necessarily part of what one does the "gamete sources" must give voluntary and informed consent "for any disposition of their embryos," but they neglect the distinction between creation that embraces destruction and employment where creation has another rationale. Nothing they say about "respect" strictly forbids taking the former step, as far as I can tell. If this is right, their case permits more than I do, at the end of the day. Second, my appeal to the double-sided nature of potentiality yields an account of how embryos and fetuses are similar and dissimilar that retains the following link. Like fetuses, they are not yet a self-elaborating power underway. Meyer and Nelson approach this account but then draw back from it. They hold that embryos are not yet "effectively a stage in the early development of a person." I accept their "effectively," if it means "not now a self-elaborating

power underway." But then they add: "Put differently, an extracorporeal embryo—whether used in research, discarded, or kept frozen—is simply not a precursor to any ongoing personal narrative. An embryo properly starts on that trajectory only when the gamete sources intentionally have it placed in a womb" (18). This is a distinct appraisal; it is not the same point "put differently." I take embryos to be the precursors to any ongoing personal narrative by virtue of the genetic properties they already have. Implantation does not create these properties or start the "trajectory" that only these properties make possible. It allows them to develop "properly." Thus, it seems more cogent to take conception and all that it alone makes possible as the point at which one should ascribe a judgment of irreducible value, for once conceived, each entity is a form of primordial human life.

33. For my subsequent account of the "nothing is lost" principle, I owe a great debt to John Reeder's volume *Killing and Saving: Abortion, Hunger, and War* and to his detailed comments on an earlier draft of this chapter.

34. This question was helpfully posed to me by Gilbert Meilaender in correspondence.

35. Reeder, *Killing and Saving,* 62–63.

36. See Baruch Brody, *Abortion and the Sanctity of Human Life: A Philosophical View* (Cambridge, Mass.: MIT Press, 1976), 151.

37. Conversations with Richard Fern shed light on the matter I raise in this paragraph, and on much else besides.

38. Sondra Wheeler led me to see that the normative position I defend requires a critical assessment of *in vitro* fertilization as currently practiced in the United States, and I thank her for perceptive counsel.

39. This position stands closer to the guidelines that the Canadian Institutes of Health Research released in March 2002 than to the more restrictive policies of the United States and the more permissive policies of the United Kingdom. "In Canada, publicly funded researchers can derive and study pluripotent human stem cell lines from embryos, fetal tissue, amniotic fluid, the umbilical cord, placenta, and somatic tissues (either from persons or cadavers). . . . Research not eligible for public funding will include studies involving the creation of clones for further research or for reproductive purposes, research involving the creation of embryos strictly for research purposes, and research in which non-human stem cells are combined with a human embryo or fetus" (see Françoise Baylis, "Canada Announces Restrictions on Publicly Funded Stem Cell Research," *Hastings Center Report,* vol. 32, no 2 [2002]: 6).

PART TWO

Embryos

FOUR

Does the Human Embryo Have a
Moral Status?

BRENT WATERS

The title of this essay is admittedly awkward. The more customary phrasing would be *What is* the moral status of the human embryo? But, as I will try to demonstrate, the customary phrasing is problematic because, in light of the contemporary nature of public moral deliberation, any eventual answer must exclude normative claims or convictions. In other words, the moral status of the human embryo is *assigned* in response to procedural considerations rather than *reflecting* an ontological standing or intrinsic value.

Pondering the moral significance of the human embryo is not a new activity. Theologians and philosophers, for instance, have pondered the perennially vexing issue of when something like a "soul" animates or is present in the human body. Augustine remained uncertain whether a soul was present in a fetus that dies in its mother's womb,[1] whereas Thomas Aquinas asserted that a soul is present at an unspecified point following conception.[2] Neither is there any agreement among modern writers, whose views range from a soul being integral with a living human body at any stage of its development[3] to an emergent soul dependent on certain minimal levels of cerebral function[4] to its irrelevance for religious belief and practice.[5] Nor is any greater theological or philosophical consensus achieved when the term "person" is exchanged for "soul," because there is bitter contention over what characteristics constitute personhood.[6]

Although contemplating the moral significance of the human embryo is not a new issue, we are now attempting to discern this significance within a novel set of circumstances. Unlike previous generations, we may now create embryos for the *sole* purpose of conducting scientific experiments, presumably to enable the development of more efficacious medical treatments. It is important that we come to terms with the sheer novelty of this capability, for it seemingly requires us to strip away the procreative contexts in which we have traditionally thought about our responsibilities in relation to the embryo. In light of this capability, for example, the notion of a parental relationship and its accompanying duties is rendered irrelevant.

Yet in stripping away this procreative context, are we not also abstracting the human embryo out from the very setting in which its meaning and worth may be discerned? If we entertain the possibility that an embryo may be created without any intention of implanting it in a womb, what exactly is this "entity" or "object" that we are beholding and whose fate we are contemplating? Or, perhaps more importantly, why do we believe that focusing our deliberation on an abstracted embryo will help us discern more clearly its moral status?

Moral Thresholds?

In answer to these questions, we are endeavoring to establish a threshold somewhat along the following lines: when an embryo reaches a certain point of development as determined by its manifesting certain characteristics, it is granted a moral status that it did not possess previously. In setting this developmental threshold, we may follow the U.K. lead of fourteen days. At this point, twinning may no longer occur, thereby creating a second embryo, and it is also at this stage that the primitive streak first appears. But more or less restrictive points along the developmental scale, such as six days for the ability to implant in a womb or twenty-eight days for the onset of a heartbeat, could also be employed as markers.[7] Prior to reaching whatever point is set, it would be permissible to do such things as harvest stem cells or clone an embryo, but, on reaching the developmental point where a moral status is attained, these same acts would be forbidden.

It must be emphasized, however, that no ontological or normative claims about the human embryo per se are being made or evoked in setting this moral status. Attaining the prescribed developmental threshold (be it six, fourteen, or twenty-eight days) does not indicate that an embryo now has a soul or is a person. If this were the case, certain binding moral rules, duties, or obligations would presumably be extended to *all* embryos. Such a moral status, however, would virtually prohibit aborting fetuses beyond the developmental threshold, unless a far less restrictive marker (such as twenty-four weeks for viability or thirty-six weeks for birth) was used as the criterion for conducting research. Yet employing this criterion would defeat the purpose for establishing the embryo's moral status, namely, to assuage the fears of a squeamish public that no one will be harmed in conducting this research—at least within a laboratory.

The latest quest to establish *the* moral status of the embryo, then, is one confined to the laboratory, and the end of this quest is not to discover the embryo's inherent ontological or normative standing, but a procedural standard enabling us to pursue potentially beneficial research in a politically palatable manner: thus the need to establish a restrictive threshold that does not in turn impinge on the reproductive rights of individuals to either terminate a pregnancy or to seek technological assistance in obtaining a child. Ironically, the human embryo is abstracted out from a procreative context, presumably to encourage deliberation on its moral status in a more objective manner, in light of the technological capability that is now at our disposal. Yet we discover that such an attempt at objectivity is trumped by the stubborn reality that it is, after all, the differing contexts of a laboratory or a woman's body, as well as the differing purposes for which embryos are created within the boundaries of these contexts, that will determine the fate of a particular embryo.

The practical effect of attempting to determine the moral status of an abstract embryo is that this status—or, better, its value—will be assigned by whoever *owns* the embryo. The concept of embryo as property that can be owned and disposed of as such should not prove startling. The advent of reproductive technology has already paved the way for this type of thinking, for in order to justify its various and often contradictory uses, we have been forced to reinterpret what procreation and parenthood now mean. Becoming a parent designates the successful culmination of, to use Gilbert Meilaender's apt depiction, a reproductive project.[8] This image accords well with the presently dominant language of reproductive freedom or procreative liberty. According to its leading proponent, the basic tenet of this doctrine is that every person has a fundamental right to either reproduce or refrain from reproducing.[9] Persons choosing to reproduce should have the freedom to employ whatever technological assistance they require to exercise this right. Individuals pursuing their reproductive interests are portrayed as "commissioners" who are free to negotiate with willing "collaborators" in providing whatever gametes or gestational services might be required. Moreover, so long as the terms of these reproductive contracts are followed, no one is harmed in these collaborative projects, because embryos lack the requisite character-istics—such as autonomy and an interest in how they should be treated—to be regarded as persons.

A subtle, though highly significant, shift in emphasis must be noted in this portrayal of procreation. Parenthood is no longer perceived, at least ideally, as the fruition of an intimate and embodied relationship between a woman and a man. Rather, parenthood signifies an act of will that is asserted through the means of various combinations of natural and technological channels. Parents are those individuals who commission and direct a reproductive proj-ect toward the successful outcome of obtaining a child. Most importantly, *all* reproductive pursuits are reduced to collaborative projects. The only dif-ference, for example, between a fertile married couple conceiving and bear-ing a child naturally and an infertile man requiring donated gametes and a surrogate mother is the scope of the collaboration required in achieving the identical end of obtaining a child.

Conceiving parenthood exclusively as an act of will implies, however, that the resulting embryo is an artifact of that will, and an artifact connotes a strong sense of property whose various uses are assigned by its owner. An em-bryo is, both figuratively and literally, willed into being by its commissioners, who in turn determine whether it will be allowed an opportunity for fur-ther development or discarded or used for other purposes if not needed. The advent of reproductive technology, when joined with an ethic of reproduc-tive freedom, has already gone a long way toward abstracting the embryo out from a procreative setting, thereby enabling us to contemplate its so-called moral status within alternative contexts in which varying values may be as-signed. Consequently, individuals producing embryos for the purpose of ob-taining a child will assign (at least some) embryos a value affording them a wide range of protections, whereas those creating embryos for the purpose of conducting research will assign a value resulting in few, if any, protections.

Posing the question of the embryo's moral status *in light of* its potential to enable the development of beneficial medical treatments presupposes that it will be answered in such a way that its assigned value will not impede re-search while also not preventing individuals from pursuing their reproduc-tive interests. The only real issue at stake is establishing a relatively restrictive or permissive procedural threshold that all but the most extreme interest groups could endorse or at least tolerate. If this were not the case, then we would also be required to revisit the moral status of embryos in the womb, as well as the infertility clinic, nor could we attempt to maintain the dubious distinction between so-called reproductive and therapeutic cloning. But we need not do the former and can accomplish the latter precisely because we already know that we are pondering the embryo within a new scientific and medical context whose status or value must thereby be assigned accordingly.

What is most troubling in trying to preserve some semblance of respect for the human embryo within the laboratory by assigning it an abstract moral status is that we may, ironically, propel ourselves down a road where we will come to perceive the human body as little more than a collection of biological commodities whose malleable value will be determined largely by rapidly shifting markets of medical goods and services. If, for instance, we should come to impose a relatively restrictive threshold for conducting embryonic research, would we not be forced to once again determine and reassign the embryo's moral status if it were discovered that a slightly more permissive threshold might lead to even more beneficial medical advances? And, as our increased use of reproductive technology and seemingly endless disputes over abortion already indicate, we can and frequently do revisit the moral status of embryos within various contexts, assigning the corresponding changes in value with alarming regularity. Moreover, it should remain for us an at least highly questionable proposition that a moral economy encouraging the development and exchange of biological commodities is suitable for attaining the kind of human flourishing it purportedly promotes in other than the most ignoble materialist terms.

Is the Embryo My Neighbor?

In response to this prospect, I propose that we explore an alternative, or perhaps parallel, question: is the human embryo my neighbor? The principal reason why this question may offer a more promising starting point for moral deliberation is, following Karl Barth, that it is much more difficult to think about neighbors in an abstract manner.[10] We cannot contemplate a neighbor in isolation, but only in relationship to and with other neighbors. We cannot even imagine what human life would be like in the absence of neighbors, for they are a ubiquitous characteristic of our individual lives and our common life. We have neighbors near and far. There are neighbors we know and neighbors we have never met. We have neighbors who are our friends and neighbors who are our enemies. Moreover, when encountering unfamiliar neighbors, we presume, or at least should presume, that we share a mutual bond by the fact that we both exist, however qualitatively different that existence might prove to be. In short, in order to learn what being human means requires that we treat our fellow human beings as neighbors, and we must always remember that this treatment is predicated on God's command that we love our neighbors, whoever they might be.

There are two principal objections that can be raised against this alternative proposal. First, it may be objected that attempting to regard the embryo as a neighbor is too fanciful to be of much practical use. We cannot seriously treat embryos *as if* they are our neighbors, because we cannot interact or form relationships with them. To regard the embryo as a neighbor would require an imaginative leap that most reasonable people could not be expected to achieve.

Being a good neighbor, however, does not always require reciprocity or even interaction. We are quite capable of protecting nameless and vulnerable neighbors, even assisting those we never meet or directly encounter as demonstrated by our acts of kindness and charity. Regarding embryos as our neighbor requires, admittedly, an imaginative leap on our part, but this prospect should not in itself prevent us from undertaking the intellectual challenge. Previous generations must have surely felt daunted in their initial attempts to include more fully, for instance, women, children, and slaves within the range of their moral vision, yet most of us today would judge their efforts to leap these chasms as altogether good and righteous endeavors. Moreover, at the very time when serious proposals are being issued, urging us to perceive the treatment of animals within an expanded sphere of friendship, it is surely not all that fanciful to regard human embryos within a realm of neighborliness.[11] If we can entertain the possibility of treating an animal as a friend, is it really an unimaginable stretch to regard an embryo as a neighbor?

Second, it may be objected that attempting to regard embryos as neighbors will only lead to an equally abstract form of moral deliberation, thereby eliminating the very rationale for my alternative approach. The history of an ethic of neighbor-love does not have a very promising record for preserving the particularity of the objects of moral reflection that I seemingly wish to preserve in grieving the loss of a procreative context. Indeed, a disinterested neighbor-love has generated the concept of *equal regard* that makes all neighbors, whoever they might be, little more than highly abstract collections of conflicting interests and duties. In late modernity, these conflicts are often resolved by thin justifications for the strong asserting their will over the weak. The proposed thresholds within the laboratory I decry would at least afford these embryos some minimal protection from the most grievous exploitation.

Admittedly, the momentum of a love-for-neighbor ethic will be difficult to overcome, but it is not an impossible task. We may deliberate on our responsibilities to neighbors, whoever they may be, without *necessarily* abstracting them in a disinterested manner. We may conceive these responsibilities within concentric spheres of love that take into account the particular or special obligations that occur, for example, in the relationship between children and parents. An account of neighbor-love stressing the particular nature of this intergenerational relationship might serve as a reminder that we share with an embryo an underlying equality before God, and the neighbor we encounter at this stage of development *is* little more than a mass of cells. Moreover, regardless of how thin the moral justifications have become, the overriding principle of an ethic of neighbor-love has remained the protection of the weak and innocent. Rather than jettisoning this principle in light of growing technological and medical potential, the range of moral regard has simply constricted to focus on the neighbor as autonomous person rather than the neighbor as dependent human being. Thus, a more robust, particularistic, and expansive explication of neighbor-love may also serve to indict late modernity's impoverished moral vision, especially in light of a greater technological potential to exploit, should the scope of moral regard be restricted even more tightly.

I acknowledge, however, that regarding the embryo as neighbor will not make the task of pondering its fate any less demanding. Indeed, with respect to conducting research, it will probably make the task of obeying God's command to love our neighbors all the more perplexing. There are no easy or obvious choices to be made when the needs, obligations, and limitations of *all* the neighbors involved are taken into account.

We cannot casually or curtly dismiss, for instance, the possibility that for many individuals embryonic stem cell research represents the best, perhaps only, hope for effectively treating a severely debilitating injury or mortal illness. Providing effective medical care is a powerful expression of love for these neighbors in need. Using our scientific knowledge and medical skill to help the lame walk, the blind see, and the deaf hear remains a faithful witness to Christ the healer.[12] It is arguable that to withhold or refuse to develop treatments that might restore health is, prima facie, an act of bad faith against these needful neighbors. It is, after all, the Samaritan who stopped and actually treated the wounds of the beaten man who proved to be the good neighbor.[13]

Nevertheless, although ameliorating suffering is a genuine sign of neighbor-love, its expression is not without limit nor must it be implemented at any cost. The very love that calls us to alleviate suffering is the same love that also requires us to protect the weakest and most vulnerable neighbor. Thus, we may, under certain circumstances, be required to sacrifice our own interests and well-being, or even compel others to forgo certain benefits, for the sake of powerless neighbors. It is in lifting up this sacrificial dimension of neighbor-love that we bear a faithful witness to Christ the suffering servant.

It is also precisely the fluidity of this sacrificial dimension that enables us to regard the embryo as neighbor, thereby preventing us from simply defining it out of our moral vision. It is the state of a being's needfulness, weakness, or vulnerability that commands our moral regard as neighbor *and not* the characteristics of the being who happens to be needful, weak, or vulnerable. Or, following George Grant, we must ever keep before us the fact that the embryo on whose fate we are deliberating is alive and not inert and is human and not something else.[14] There is a generic and given bond among humans, regardless of their relative stages of development, by virtue of their shared biology, that is more adequately captured in a presumption of neighborliness than that of something like personhood. Without this generic presumption, it becomes all too easy to simply disregard specialized categories of humans because they are not persons or they exist in an inherently inferior stage of development. Thus, the idea of sacrificing one's interest for the sake of an embryo is rendered unintelligible. Yet simply to define the human embryo out from our moral regard is merely to devise a tidy rationalization for the most crass exploitation, a strategy used all too often and effectively in the past to justify exploiting "inherently inferior" humans such as women and slaves. It is in virtue of an embryo's given status as *human* that the possibility of sacrificing one's interest for the sake of this neighbor becomes intelligible.

It must be admitted, however, that recapturing this intelligibility does not necessarily prohibit using embryos for the purpose of research, even if it results in their willful destruction. If neighbor-love is to avoid becoming a hollow ethic of equal regard, we must also acknowledge that there is a hierarchy of duties and obligations that we owe to different types of neighbors. Not all neighbors are the same, requiring identical regard and treatment on our part. And although the contexts in which we encounter these varying neighbors are not solely determinative for how we should regard and treat them, they do go a long way in shaping a fitting moral vision and its requisite acts.

Thus, we must at least be open to the possibility that there are those rare occasions when we may conclude that certain neighbors (such as weak and vulnerable embryos) may be sacrificed because of the genuine needs of other (ill
or injured) neighbors. The question we are now called to deliberate on is if
the technological potential to utilize human embryos in developing new and
efficacious medical treatments is one of these rare occasions.

I conclude this essay with a confession: I remain ambivalent about the
prospect of human embryonic stem cell research. On the one hand, I recognize the potential benefits this research might produce. I take seriously the
proposition that medical care is a profoundly moral act of expressing a genuine love for needful neighbors. Moreover, as a Christian I believe we are
called to use medicine to do more than merely keep company with those
who suffer. On the other hand, although I have argued elsewhere that conducting research on embryos is permissible within a highly attenuated set of
parameters, I am deeply troubled by the latest proposals.[15] I also take seriously
the possibility that this research is being driven by a technical rationality that
has so badly warped our moral vision that we have now started haphazardly
toward a destination we may very well regret. As a Christian, I am particularly alarmed at how quickly and easily late moderns have already constricted
the range of their moral regard in accommodating every so-called medical
and technological advance.

It is no doubt due to this ambivalence that my thinking about the human
embryo also remains untidy. As I hope I have demonstrated, I have little confidence that setting a threshold for establishing a moral status for the human
embryo will do anything more than justify tentative and relatively aggressive research protocols. We will simply purchase a clean conscience by de-
luding ourselves that no one, at least no one of any real significance, will be
harmed in this research. I hope I have also demonstrated that, although conceiving the human embryo as a neighbor might add a richer and deeper dimension to public moral deliberation, it does not make the task of discernment any easier. But if we choose to go down the road of a research project
that many assure us will result in unprecedented advances in health care, I
would at least prefer to make that journey in the company of embryos I regard as neighbors rather than as abstract objects to which I must assign a value
or moral status.

Acknowledgments

I am indebted to Andy Watts and Tripp York, for their comments and criticisms of an earlier draft of this essay.

Notes

1. See Augustine, *City of God* XXII/13.

2. See Thomas Aquinas, *Summa Theologica* Ia, q.92.

3. See, e.g., Germain Grisez, *The Way of the Lord Jesus* II (Quincy, Ill.: Franciscan Press, 1993), 464–67, and J. P. Moreland and Scott B. Rae, *Body and Soul: Human Nature and the Crisis in Ethics* (Downers Grove, Ill.: InterVarsity Press, 2000), 199–228.

4. See, e.g., Richard Swinburne, *The Evolution of the Soul* (Oxford: Clarendon Press, 1986).

5. See, e.g., Joseph Fletcher, *Morals and Medicine* (Boston: Beacon Press, 1960), 216–18.

6. There is a voluminous literature regarding theological and philosophical accounts of personhood. For a summary of the principal issues at stake, particularly in respect to bioethics, see H. Tristram Engelhardt, Jr., *The Foundations of Bioethics* (New York: Oxford University Press, 1996), 135–88.

7. See James C. Peterson, *Genetic Turning Points: The Ethics of Human Genetic Intervention* (Grand Rapids, Mich.: Eerdmans, 2001), 117–34.

8. See Gilbert Meilaender, *Bioethics: A Primer for Christians* (Grand Rapids, Mich.: Eerdmans, 1996), 11–25. See also Oliver O'Donovan, *Begotten or Made?* (Oxford: Clarendon Press, 1984), 1–13.

9. See John A. Robertson, *Children of Choice: Freedom and the New Reproductive Technologies* (Princeton, N.J.: Princeton University Press, 1994). For theological critiques of Robertson, see Gilbert C. Meilaender, *Body, Soul, and Bioethics* (Notre Dame, Ind.: University of Notre Dame Press, 1995), 61–88, and Brent Waters, *Reproductive Technology: Towards a Theology of Procreative Stewardship* (Cleveland: Pilgrim Press, 2001), 19–22.

10. See Karl Barth, *Church Dogmatics,* vol. 3, part 4 (Edinburgh: T & T Clark, 1961), 285–323.

11. See, e.g., Stephen Clark, *Biology and Christian Ethics* (Cambridge: Cambridge University Press, 2000).

12. See Matthew 11:2–6.

13. See Luke 10:29–37.

14. See George Grant, *Technology and Justice* (Notre Dame: University of Notre Dame Press, 1986), 120–23.

15. See Waters, *Reproductive Technology*, 102–27.

FIVE

Is a Human Embryo a Human Being?

JAMES C. PETERSON

Motivating donors, sound bites, party politics, and legislation all look for simple bright lines against moral horrors, often brighter lines of demarcation than are actually there. There are real horrors, but the division between heading toward or away from them is often difficult to discern with precision. In this brief chapter, I will not have the space to explain and defend a conclusion on the theme of this book, how God would have us treat each human embryo.[1] There will just be space here to briefly introduce and begin to test some of the most widely given reasons for protecting human embryos as people. If, in the next few pages, we can clear away some of the common but mistaken arguments about whether an embryo is or is not a person and also highlight some concerns that need further reflection, the contribution will be substantial.

One current debate centers on whether stem cells should be obtained by taking apart human embryos. I am not aware of any objection to using stem cells to help people. What is at issue is the source of stem cells. If stem cells could be obtained from inessential cells of an adult patient, we could have a perfect tissue match for the person being treated with no risk of rejection and no moral question. Such stem cells would possibly save countless lives from paralysis, Alzheimer's, Parkinson's, and other debilitating, even deadly, diseases. To find a way to do so would be a kind and fruitful expression of love for those neighbors. That is well worth pursuing. It may some day be possible, but it is not now and it will not be easy to reach if we do. Although most nucleated cells have all the genetic instructions for a complete human body, an adult cell has formed into the most effective structure for doing a specialized task. A tiny fraction of the DNA in the cell is guiding the cell's work. The information is there to make anything in the body, but the DNA and the rest of the cell have been configured for a particular task. To reform the DNA into the unshaped potential of an original stem cell is physically wrenching. Some labs have held out hope that someday we will be able to do it without damaging the information, but in the meantime, and it may be a very long time, millions of people are struggling, and many are dying, who might be helped sooner by embryonic stem cells. Should we obtain potentially life-giving stem cells from the death of embryos?

There is no problem with sacrificing human tissue to save human beings, but is the embryo more than just tissue? If the embryo is a fellow human being, we should not kill one person to save another. Human beings are simply not available to cut into parts, no matter how useful. But is an embryo the smallest of human beings, a person, a soul? News accounts of the stem cell debate have often expressed surprise that many individuals who have worked actively against abortion have been willing to accept the taking apart of early human embryos to obtain stem cells. That some prolife activists would reject one and accept the other is rooted in their understanding of what the embryo is. Some argue that, although an embryo is more than just tissue, it is not yet a person. In contrast, others argue that a human embryo, as an embryo, is already a particular human being. What does the Christian faith say about the view that a human embryo is a person or at least to be treated as such?

Most Christians over the centuries have sought to know God and God's will by listening to scripture, tradition, direct experience of God, and thoughtful reason. Different streams within the varied Christian tradition have emphasized one of these sources over another. For example, the Reformation was rooted in *sola scriptura,* but this was never scripture alone. It was rather scripture *first,* interpreted in the light of tradition, experience, and reason. I will begin with scripture.

Scripture

In Islam, the Koran simply states that a person is first present forty days after fertilization. The Christian tradition has no such clear statement. Texts such as Psalm 139:13 are often quoted. It reads, "You knit me together in my mother's womb." The metaphor of knitting conveys God's close involvement in the psalmist's life from the beginning. It does not say, however, when that form in the womb became a human being. God is intimately involved in the formation of the body that will be the psalmist. That does not tell us when the developing body *is* the psalmist. Trying indirectly to extrapolate the timing of human presence from this text is reading in affirmations that are not present.

Jeremiah 1:5 is often quoted, "Before you were in the womb I knew you, before you were born I set you apart." The text, however, is not about human embryology or even about humanity at all. It is about the surety of what God plans. God has called Jeremiah to a particular vocation and has been planning this task even before Jeremiah was in the womb. There is nothing in the text that designates when Jeremiah became a human being. If the point of the text was instruction about the start of Jeremiah's existence, it would indicate that he was alive in some realm before being in the womb. Again, the quote reads, "*Before* you were in the womb, I knew you." Preexistence is not the point any more than for Ephesians 1:4, which states that "God chose us in Him before the creation of the world." The texts are marveling at God's foreknowledge and choice, not human existence before time. God knows what is in even the secret place of the womb (Job 31:15). Embryos are in God's presence, as is all the rest of life. We are responsible for how we treat them, but when precisely they become persons is not taught in these texts.

A third text that is often cited is found in the law for the people of Israel. Exodus 21:22–23 differs markedly from one translation to another. In the New International Version (NIV) it reads, "If men who are fighting hit a pregnant woman and she gives birth prematurely but there is no serious injury, the offender must be fined whatever the woman's husband demands and the court allows. But if there is serious injury, you are to take life for life." After the phrase "gives birth prematurely" an asterisk refers one to the alternate reading "she has a miscarriage." The NIV text translation is that the fight has caused labor, but the delivered baby is healthy, hence minimal penalty is appropriate for putting the baby at risk.[2] The NIV alternative reading is that a miscarriage has been triggered, a serious offense, but not at the level of taking a human life. If a human life had been lost, the death penalty would have been required, eye for an eye, tooth for a tooth. Translation uncertainty is at precisely the point where the passage might have shed some light on the question before us. Orthodox Jews, listening to this text and other scripture with deep respect, have developed a consensus that human life should be protected beginning forty days after conception. Before that point, there is something which is human and alive, as in any human tissue, but not yet a fellow person.

Specifically Christian scripture is clear that God is aware and cares about all the stages of human life. Whereas Jesus' disciples were anxious to send away children who wanted to meet him, Jesus welcomed them. Luke uses the same word to describe the children brought to Jesus for blessing, the newborn Jesus, and the not yet born John the Baptist.[3] There is concern for all, including the most vulnerable, but the Christian scripture does not precisely address when any particular human being begins. Harold O. J. Brown, who vigorously advocates the presence of each person beginning with conception, is scrupulously honest in his careful exegesis. He admits that scripture does not directly describe the human person as being present at the time of conception.[4] Pope John Paul II, a fierce opponent of abortion, writes, "The texts of Sacred Scripture never address the question of deliberate abortion and so do not directly and specifically condemn it."[5] The Lutheran theologian Gilbert Meilaender unfailingly advocates nurture for the unborn and summarizes, "We cannot, I think, claim that the Bible itself establishes the point at which an individual life begins, although it surely directs our attention to the value of fetal life."[6]

The most relevant theme that we do have from Christian scripture is that followers of Jesus Christ should love their neighbors. Jesus describes this in Luke 10 as a concern for others that calls one to help whomever one can help. Responsibility, nurture, and service are at the fore, yet the following question remains. Granted we should love our neighbor and that we know our neighbors who are dying from disease, when is there a neighbor in the womb to love? Scripture directs us to extend our love to all our neighbors, but it does not specifically tell us when in the womb there is a neighbor present to love. We should exercise hospitality, but does that include every sperm or egg? Every conceptus? Every embryo in a petri dish? The call to love our neighbor does not in itself tell us when there is a neighbor present to love.

Tradition

We could turn to tradition, the wisdom of our brothers and sisters in the faith who have lived before us. They have thoughtfully and diligently sought to follow the same Lord. For much of church history, the dominant view of how human beings begin has been that there is not an ensouled body until there is a body to ensoul.

Through the early and medieval church, the long-standing consensus among theologians was that God gave a soul at the point when a body had formed in the womb. Or in the perspective of "traducianism," a soul seed inherited from one's parents develops with the body and is at last fully present when there is a formed body. Both soul creation and traducianism reasoned that one needed a body to have a soul, whether the soul is emergent or assigned. Before a body was present, the life developing in the womb was described as "unformed." The distinction between unformed and formed was used by early church teachers such as Tertullian, Lactantius, Jerome, Augustine in the *Enchiridion*, Cyril of Alexandria, and Theodoret.[7] Estimates as to exactly when the body was formed varied, but centered on about two months postconception. Thomas Aquinas, "the angelic doctor" of the Roman Catholic tradition, set it at precisely forty days from conception for boys and ninety days for girls. Why the different number of days for males and females? Aquinas was using what he perceived to be the best science available in his day, the numbers given by Aristotle.[8]

Church tradition saw allusions to the distinction between unformed and formed in three scriptural texts. One reference was clearest in the language chosen by the Septuagint. The Septuagint was the widely used Greek translation of the Hebrew Bible. Its translation of the Exodus 21:22–23 passage discussed earlier makes this distinction. There is a monetary penalty for ending *unformed* life, but it *formed* life is killed, the death penalty is required, life for life. Second, in the Hebrew-language scripture, human beings are often called *nephesh*, an animated body. Can one be an animated body, without a body? Granted one still has a body after a leg amputation or the removal of a cancerous kidney, but having a substantial body of some sort still remains basic to being a human being in this world. Third, in Job 10:10–11, Job prays "Did you not pour me out like milk and curdle me like cheese, then clothe me with skin and flesh and knit me together with bones and sinews?" This was read as a description of life beginning with an unformed state and then later developing to a formed one. By this distinction between unformed and formed, not yet having a body and having a body, miscarriage or abortion before formation was seen as loss of what could become a human body. Miscarriage or abortion after formation was the tragic loss of a present body and person.

To appeal to formation with our current knowledge of development might lead one to about twenty-eight days postfertilization as the time to recognize that a neighbor is present. By about that point, the fetus has a heartbeat and brain activity will soon follow. All of the major organ systems exist, with future growth coming in size and refinement. Despite recent Vatican teaching that a human being is present from conception, there is still an active discussion of the developmental tradition among Roman Catholics. Margaret Farley cites herself, Lisa Cahill, Thomas Shannon, and James J. Walter as examples of widely read theologians who, as they seek to thoughtfully carry on the Catholic tradition, see the first presence of a person at a point later than conception.[9]

Experience

We could turn to our experience of God's leading. George Annas appeals to a common moral intuition with the following story.[10] If a fire broke out in a fertility lab and there was only time to save a visiting two-month-old baby in a bassinet or a test tube rack containing seven embryos, most people would save the baby without hesitation. Yet carrying out the test tube rack instead could have saved seven people, if indeed each embryo were a person. Thankfully, that is not the usual choice that we face. But if Annas is correct about what we would do, what is guiding our choice? Could it be that we do perceive a clear distinction between an embryo as potentially a person and a later point in development as a person actually present?

Reason

Can reason resolve the question? It is often claimed that human development is a continuum and no point along it marks when a human being has begun. Hence, a human being must be present from fertilization. The irony of this argument is that it has not escaped staking out a transition point on the continuum from human life to a human person. It is still citing a point at which a person first becomes present. All of the genes that an individual has were already in the living human egg and sperm that would meet. It is bringing them together in one place that is seen as the crucial threshold. So, by this view, there is still a threshold condition for the presence of a person. It is the presence of all the genes for one person in one cell. That then raises the question of why mark the gathering of the genes for a unique individual as the crucial transition? Yes, the single microscopic fertilized cell is alive, human (since from humans), and genetically individual, but these three attributes also apply to some of the skin cells that we regularly lose without regret in daily life.

Usually the argument shifts at this point to one of potential. For the first time, at conception, there is now an organism that has all the needed genetic instructions to form a human body. Actually every nucleated human cell—3,000,000,000 in each human being—has a complete copy of these instructions. So, on this basis alone, every nucleated cell would warrant nurture and protection. We could qualify the argument that the fertilized egg can grow on its own, but that would not be true. If it is in a petri dish, it needs a woman to welcome and physically nurture it in her womb in order to survive. A fertilized egg cannot develop without extensive support. If some day all nucleated cells could be implanted and develop into individual human beings, would each of them warrant treatment as a person because of their potential as well?

Another variation on this argument says that the embryo *is* a human being because we have all been that size early in our development. A microscopic ball of identical cells is what all human beings look like at that age. Note that standing alone this statement is not so much an argument as a conclusion. All acknowledge that in the development of human life there is such a stage. The question before us is still when in that human development is a person present? There may be an implicit appeal in the assertion, that potential to develop into someone we would all recognize as a human being is the same as being a human being. But potential means not yet, if ever, not that what has potential has already become or is guaranteed to become what it has the potential to be. An acorn has the potential to become an oak tree and may or may not actually become an oak tree. There is an involved metaphysical argument that a human being is fully present as an embryo and only unfolds that presence over time, but such an argument ignores the formative role of the environment in the womb and beyond. Genes do not determine all the physical characteristics of an individual, let alone who the person will be as a person. A set of genes does not a person make. Think of identical twins with identical genes who yet become and remain unique persons. Further, even if a genetic start guaranteed a later outcome, which it does not, that does not mean what is present should be treated as what it will be. All readers of this chapter are likely to someday be corpses, but that does not mean that we should be treated as corpses now. Having the potential to become something is not the same as already being that thing.

If developing human life becomes a particular human being some time after fertilization, when might that be? Some writers and governments have seen the threshold at successful implantation about six to nine days after fertilization, because the embryo's chance of birth increases from not likely (roughly one in three) to likely. The exact proportion of embryo loss is contested, but that more than half of what is conceived never implants is clear. It can be said that infant mortality has been that high in times and places of human history and that infants are no less persons as a result. But if a person is present from conception, God's design for human beings is that a majority will never experience life on earth. Of course God could choose to do this, but it seems contrary to what has been revealed as God's plan for human beings to live and choose here. Ronald Green notes that if we are convinced that this embryo loss is the end of half of humanity in the days before implantation (a loss of human life beyond the scale of the medieval black plague), should not the greatest share of federal research money and all other available resources be devoted to saving them?[11] If half of all the people who have ever been created are lost in those first days, that is a far greater loss of life than to cancer, AIDS, or other diseases that currently attract our greatest efforts.

Others have argued that fourteen days after fertilization is the transition to the presence of a fellow human being because that is when it finally becomes clear whether the embryo actually is an individual or several people. Identical twins or triplets can spring from one embryo up to that point. Also two embryos can merge to develop into one person. For those who think a soul is assigned at conception, the biological reality of twinning would mean that either some embryos that will not survive are soulless from the beginning or some embryos carry two souls until they split. There could not be a simple one-soul-to-one-embryo correspondence from fertilization. What is highlighted in this concern is not whether there is life present. The number of lives beginning in one embryo would make no difference in that regard. It is rather taking seriously the argument that a person begins when one unique human continuum has begun. That is often associated with conception, but it is actually not settled until fourteen days after fertilization.

It should be noted that recognizing a person at implantation (six to nine days), individuation (fourteen days), or formation (twenty-eight days) is not to suggest that human beings can be more or less human according to their mastery of certain capabilities, as if being a human being was a degreed property. That would leave people with various disabilities vulnerable to being declared nonhuman. The lines described above are each proposed as thresholds. Once the threshold is crossed, the individual is a human being, whether attaining an ideal or not. It has also been suggested in a related concern that one should not even think in terms of transition from human life to person or human being, because such a focus excludes human beings who should be included. To point out that a description of human beings sees some instances of human life as not being human, however, is not an objection to such a description, it is characteristic of every definition of human beings. I am not aware of anyone who argues that each human sperm is a human being or that sloughed-off human skin cells, alive with a full complement of one individual's genes, are persons. To reject a description of what is needed to be a human being, one would need to show that someone who is a human being has been excluded, not simply that the description does not include as a human being everything that comes from humans and that is alive.

Burden of Proof

Where each side claims justification from the same concern is in burden of proof. One side argues that we should not take a chance on ending a human embryo's life because a person *might* be present. If there is any chance that a person may be present, that possibility should receive every protection. Proponents of using embryos for stem cell research appeal to the burden of proof as well. They say that we know there are undeniably people dying of diabetes, Parkinson's, Alzheimer's, congestive heart failure, and other diseases who could be helped by replacing lost tissue. Painful and chronic diseases such as osteoarthritis and rheumatoid arthritis might be helped by replacement therapy as well. Most stem cells in the body produce only certain differentiated cells. It may be possible to coax them into forming other needed tissue, but only undifferentiated embryonic stem cells clearly have the ability to develop any human tissue. Although such therapy is not available at the time of this book's printing, lives may one day be saved by embryonic stem cells. How can we let patients who are unmistakably people die to protect embryos that, even if implanted, may or may not turn out to someday become persons? We should not kill people to benefit others, but we should also not let people die to protect human tissue such as sperm or ova, even though such gametes do have great potential. Has the connection of one sperm and one egg together now made present a human being, who, as a human being, should of course not be sacrificed? Notice, each side sees the burden of proof argument as favoring its conclusion. Both are concerned about loving our neighbors, particularly those in great need. One advocates possible help for identified persons. The other identified help for possible persons. For both sides, deciding either way is a matter of life and death for many human beings.

A variation of the burden of proof argument is that, if any developing human life is not nurtured, we will slide down a slippery slope into the kind of horrific slaughter perpetrated by the Nazis. This concern refers both to a conceptual slippery slope that, once it is acceptable to kill one human life, there is no longer a clear prohibition to refrain from killing many, and a social slippery slope that, even if there is a good reason to stop abortion at an early stage of pregnancy, the societal momentum of allowing early abortion will be such that we will not stop any abortion. Such has indeed been the experience of the United States since *Roe v. Wade*. Abortion is now allowed up to the time of birth, and there are prominent ethicists who currently argue for infanticide. The slippery slope argument concludes that human beings need protection beginning at some clear early threshold or they will eventually not be protected at all. Slippery slope concerns are well worth considering. They are compelling to the degree that there is a slippery slope and the end to which it leads is abhorred. Middle positions have been proposed in response that the clear line to be drawn does not have to be at fertilization and that, even if the embryo is not a person yet, the embryo could still as a human embryo warrant more respect and care than mere tissue. Such a status might still offer good reasons to protect embryos, just not at the near absolute level that they would warrant as people.

This chapter has focused on one important aspect of the questions before us. Is a human embryo a fellow human being? Of course there is more to consider than could be tested in these few pages, but I hope this chapter has given good reasons to put aside some of the rhetoric that has obscured more than helped and highlighted some of the arguments calling for more attention. Recognizing the status of human embryos is central to crucial decisions that will only increase in number and import. Even if effective stem cells can someday be obtained from sources other than embryos, the status of human embryos will still make a difference for somatic cell nuclear transfer, preimplantation genetic diagnosis, and a myriad of other present and future techniques. To think clearly about the human embryo and then treat it appropriately will continue to require our best attention.

Notes

1. My recent book, *Genetic Turning Points: The Ethics of Human Genetic Intervention* (Grand Rapids, Mich.: Eerdmans, 2001), has the space to address a wider range of the involved concerns from our relation with nature to the risk of commodifying children.

2. John Jefferson Davis succinctly lays out and evaluates three possible readings in *Abortion and the Christian: What Every Believer Should Know* (Phillipsburg, N.J.: Presbyterian & Reformed, 1984), 49–52.

3. Luke 1:41, 44, 2:12, 16, 18:15.

4. Harold O. J. Brown, as quoted by John Jefferson Davis, *Evangelical Ethics: Issues Facing the Church Today* (Phillipsburg, N.J.: Presbyterian and Reformed, 1985), 148.

5. Pope John Paul II, *Evangelium Vitae* (The Gospel of Life) (New York: Random House, 1995), 108.

6. Gilbert Meilaender, *Bioethics: A Primer for Christians* (Carlisle, U.K.: Paternoster, 1996), 29.

7. John Connery, *Abortion: The Development of the Roman Catholic Perspective* (Chicago: Loyola University Press, 1977), 40, 50–52, 56.

8. Aristotle, *On the History of Animals,* book. 7, chap. 3. There are many translations available, for example by D'Arcy Wentworth Thompson, *The Works of Aristotle,* vol. 3 (Chicago: William Benton/Encyclopedia Britannica, 1952), 108–9.

9. Margaret A. Farley, "Roman Catholic Views on hES Cell Research," in *The Human Embryonic Stem Cell Debate,* edited by Suzanne Holland, Karen Lebacqz, and Laurie Zoloth (Cambridge, Mass.: MIT Press, 2001), 115–17.

10. As quoted by Bonnie Steinbock, in *Life before Birth: The Moral and Legal Status of Embryos and Fetuses* (New York: Oxford University Press, 1992), 215.

11. Ronald M. Green, "Determining Moral Status," *American Journal of Bioethics,* vol. 2, no. 1 (winter 2002): 26.

SIX

Principles and Politics: Beyond the Impasse over the Embryo

RONALD COLE-TURNER

As one who believes that embryo research should be permitted but carefully regulated and limited, reflecting on this debate brings me to two observations. First, it does not appear at all likely that Christians, at least, will ever agree on a theological and moral assessment of the human embryo or even that a strong majority position will emerge. On the contrary, our divisions in this matter are so deep that it is hard to imagine our finding a consensus view about what the human embryo is and what we owe it.

Of course, there will be shifts in opinion in the general public and surely among Christians as well. At the moment, it may be that opinion is turning against the moral acceptability of embryo research. The National Bioethics Council has proposed a four-year moratorium on this research, in part to allow time for the arguments to be made and tested in the public arena. It is even possible that, in a few years, opinions will shift so decidedly as to provide a wide enough basis for a ban on embryo research in the United States, one that is both permanent and generally supported, for instance by legislators of both parties.

But even so, there will be a significant minority in dissent, not just among the researchers who want to do the work, but also among patients who think they are being denied treatments. And if in fact the tide of opinion is now in favor of stopping embryo research, those who favor this side should not congratulate themselves too soon. They should expect that the outcome of the public controversy might have more to do in the end with public relations than with principled argument, more in fact with our personal health anxieties or financial concerns than with moral convictions. If so, then those with the resources to wage the more effective public relations campaign or to play on our anxieties are the more likely to claim the majority in the end. So I expect the present shift (if indeed there is one) in public opinion against embryo research will turn before long toward support of research, if for no other reason because there is no money in protecting the embryo. As one who favors a limited form of this research, I have to say now that I would regret very much winning the public for the wrong reasons—on the basis of health anxieties, medical expediency, or the prospect of commercial bene-fit—or by means of the wrong methods—where the public is manipulated, not persuaded. For surely, if these are the reasons that underlie the public's eventual acceptance of embryo research, then some of the worst fears of the critics of the research will be realized, and we will demean ourselves and our society with the embryo.

The second observation is that those who oppose embryo research offer a better moral argument than do those of us who would permit it. It is un-comfortable to admit this, and it may be the nature of what they are required to argue rather than the competence of those who make the argument that explains the difference, but theirs is the more clear and straightforward case, and perhaps the easier one to make. In fact, there may be an interesting irony that will emerge here; it may prove easier to argue with rational clarity against embryo research than to win the public relations campaign against it.

How can the critics of research win against televised images of desperately sick people, images of our future selves with Alzheimer's or Parkinson's dis-ease, with such yearnings for treatments that we will come to see any cost as trivial? On the other hand, though, how can we who favor research readily counter the challenge posed in their question: if not at conception, then just when does a developing human life cross a threshold into sharing our com-mon human status and dignity? Or how do we answer their protest, with its echoes of biblical prophesy drawing on words attributed to none other than Jesus (Matt. 25), that precisely because the embryo is the least of all humans, it is most deserving of protection? By comparison, our answers are vague, poor in clarity, and devoid of prophecy.

Biology and Moral Status

Yes, of course, they have a point: conception is one of the "bright lines" of human development. But so is birth, and it is not the brightness of the line that commands our recognition of value or status as much as a careful and informed assessment of the actual state of the developing organism. When the psalmist praises God, saying, "Thou didst knit me together in my mother's womb," it is a process of formation that is being described. The text continues: "My frame was not hidden from thee, when I was being made in secret, intricately wrought in the depths of the earth" (Psalm 139:13–14). As little as biblical writers understood fetal development, they did in fact recognize that there is a "being made" here. Today, in our era of genetic determinism, when we ascribe all power to genes, we too readily ascribe ultimacy to conception, as if the fixing of our genes fixes our identity. Geneticists themselves know the depth of the error here, but too many of us persist nonetheless in allowing genetic determinism to serve as the unchallenged warrant for an argument about the exaggerated importance of conception among developmental milestones.

The trouble is that our biological development is subtle and gradual, but morality wants clarity and sometimes forces it where biology does not permit us to find it. It is better to recognize that, biologically, the overwhelming portion of our human development is gradual. It is not characterized by well-marked developmental break points, like conception or birth, that clearly mark the boundary between before and after. We must perform our moral assessment of human development in view of the reality of our gradual development. There is no clear and clean developmental break point or bright line occurring between human conception and birth. Nevertheless we can see, can we not, that the embryo *is not* a child, that something profound and momentous occurs along that precarious but gradual pathway to life. Although we cannot point out distinct mileposts in the pathway, we have no doubt at all about its reality and its profound significance for what we are.

In contrast to the certainty and clarity with which our opponents declare that the embryo is one of us *from conception*, the best we can do is say that *somewhere* between conception and birth development occurs, and through it human status emerges. *Somewhere* is a painfully vague word when pressed into this debate, but it is the right and only word to describe what is by definition a *process*. We know that, at the end of the process, the developing life is one of us. We know that, at the beginning, it is not. And we know that there is no precise moment in the process when the embryo becomes a baby.

Let us freely admit here that the line drawn at fourteen days after fertilization is nothing more than a line that is drawn on nature, not one that is found in nature. Finding it there and not, say, at day ten or twenty is of course to be explained by the usual references to the emergence of the primitive streak, the end of the possibility of twinning, and implantation in ordinary pregnancy, all of which occur somewhere around this time in the embryo's development and which, taken together, are often thought to signify individuality. Being able to explain why the line is at fourteen days and not ten or twenty, however, is not the same as justifying the line in the first place, and all we seem to be able to do is explain the line without giving it the sort of defense that we would like. None of these transitions in the life of the early embryo, even taken together, are ontologically sufficient to justify the claim that we find here a threshold between "not yet one of us" and "one of us," much less between mere cells and a human person.

This admission does not mean that there is no significance in this line, merely that its significance lies, first of all, in its social and political usefulness as a surprising point of consensus, hardly a trivial matter in this new and contentious debate. Not all, but most, of us who would permit limited embryo research would do so only to fourteen days. The social value of the line is not that it is a finding of biology, much less a conclusion of metaphysics or moral theology, but that it is an international point of agreement around which harmonized policies might be formed. But, more important, we recognize that the fourteen-day limit is a marker placed sufficiently early in embryological development that we can be sure that, developmentally considered, the embryo is so profoundly unlike us that it cannot be one of us. On what day does it become like us and therefore one of us? We cannot tell, but we can identify a point (at fourteen days) at which we can be sure that the overwhelming portion of the human developmental process has not yet even begun. Although we must not overlook the intricacies of its embryonic structure, about which we are learning more all the time, we must see nevertheless that this structure is that of an embryo, not a child, whose "being made" lies ahead of it.

Nor can we say with certainty or precision what moral status or value an embryo has at any particular day of its development. What we can say is that, until fourteen days, the developing embryo assuredly does not yet require of us that we regard it as a child, even though it does command greater respect than do ordinary cells and tissues. All our moral intuitions suggest this, and an understanding of developmental biology that is not unduly tilted toward genetic determinism confirms these intuitions that a child is one thing and an embryo quite another. We cannot find a precise line that distinguishes between "embryo" and "child," as if we could imagine that it is an embryo at one moment and fully a child at the next. But we can be sure that its becoming a child occurs later than fourteen days, and so once again the four-teen-day limit functions very well as a conservatively placed marker.

Such respect as the embryo commands—more than cells and tissues but less than a child—calls for a level of protection greater than that required for human tissues but less than that given to a child. What this means precisely depends in part on the biological and social context in which the embryo is created and exists. For instance, an embryo created naturally but not yet im-planted or known to those who conceived it stands in a different social and biological relationship to human beings than one created by in vitro fertil-ization for reproduction or one created in vitro or by cloning for research and perhaps some day for therapy, perhaps even to save the life of the one from whom it is cloned. Just what these social, biological, and technological differences mean to us religiously and morally and in terms of research pol-icy remains to be seen. About all that is clear for now is that this question requires more work. My sense is that in every case we are talking here about an embryo, even if its social, biological, and technological relationships may be different from that of another embryo at the same developmental stage and even if its biological potential or social possibility for life is low to the point of being nonexistent. In spite of these contingencies, they stand be-fore us as embryos, and if so we should treat them in morally similar ways in each of their settings.

Some critics of embryo research suggest that the human embryo is the least of all human beings and therefore the most deserving of respect. But the embryo is clearly *not* among those included in Matthew 25 or anywhere in the biblical moral or prophetic writings. Jesus specifically mentions the sick, the hungry, the unclothed, and the imprisoned—in other words, the de-prived, those from whom the goods of life are taken away. Some supporters of embryo research have suggested that this text puts the sick in a privileged position morally and therefore requires that we pursue embryo research for their benefit. Of course, we are obliged to care for the sick and even to pur-sue research for their sake, but this reply misses the point. For the critics of research, the embryo is one of us, and by its nature the least among us, always to be protected and never to be sacrificed for the benefit of another, no mat-ter how needy. For them, Matthew 25 and similar injunctions to love our neighbor or to take care of the "least" among us *include the embryo.* Our reply here should be simply that there is nothing at all in the relevant biblical texts to suggest this inclusion. As much as it might appeal to our sentiments to think embryos are included, a rigorous biblical ethic cannot support this argument.

Beneath our Disagreements

This is not to say, of course, that one might not have other reasons for believing the embryo is "one of us," as most of the critics of embryo research believe. I do not agree with them, but I am not at all sure what I can say that will persuade them to change their minds. Perhaps our difference rests in moral intuition that is beyond or beneath argument, more at the level of axiom than conclusion, and in fact we disagree here not about *what to do* but about *how to see*. When we look at the embryo, when we watch it divide and behold in wonder as it becomes a cluster of cells with the potential, if implanted, to become a fully developed human being, what is it we are seeing? What if anything lies prior to our moral vision itself so that it determines how we will see this cluster of cells? Those who look at an embryo and see a person—are they better people than the rest of us? Are they more noble and generous, or merely more sentimental and simple-minded than we? Do they know more biology, and if so does that help inform their judgment so as to explain the difference between us? In other words, how do we account for this deep and perplexing conflict of opinion?

I ask this as a Christian who is increasingly exasperated by my disagreements with other Christians. Do we disagree because they are better Christians than I, more filled with altruistic love and more able to see as Christ sees? Are they more faithful to historic Christianity, or merely behind the times? Am I living my faith with courage in the present, or am I merely and predictably a liberal Protestant, more in agreement with Judaism than with other forms of Christianity, perhaps too accepting of modernity on its own terms and too comfortable in this world to discern another? Not knowing why we disagree, I am not hopeful about our coming to agreement.

What then? Shall we Christians allow our theological impasse to stand, and do we let it be used by powerful and sometimes nonreligious forces to reinforce the American political stalemate over embryo research policy? There are other positions out there, most notably the view that the embryo is essentially a ball of cells worthy of special study but not special protection, and such positions may yet win the day. Those holding this view want to keep research unregulated and would like to see U.S. federal funding become available to support it.

For our part, however, we Christians in the United States are divided over whether the embryo deserves absolute or limited protection. Absolute respect for the embryo (that is, regarding it as the moral equivalent of a human child) translates into a public policy of a permanent ban on embryo research and presumably on many, if not all, of the practices of reproductive medicine. A position of limited respect, contingent on the state of the embryo and the early position it occupies on the path between conception and birth, translates into a policy of limited protection. This position is usually characterized by support for federal oversight and regulation of all forms of embryo research, private or publicly funded, perhaps reaching as far as imposing a new burden of oversight on the creation and use of embryos in reproductive medicine.

The political stalemate over the embryo, reaching in 2002 all the way to the conflict between the president and members of his own party in the U.S. Senate, means that for now privately funded embryo research goes forward with no restriction or oversight or even public awareness. This should please no one who holds a view of respect for the embryo, limited or absolute. For now, embryos may not only be created by any means and used for any purpose in most of the states in the United States, but the knowledge of this research is not even available to the public unless the researchers should choose to publish their results or file a patent application. What does anyone expect from this situation but that in time, as the results of embryo research are occasionally reported in the scientific literature and in the general media, and as the publicists for this research proclaim the wonders of its benefits, the public in general will become first complacent, then accepting, then supportive? Or could it be (and is this not equally plausible) that some corporate laboratory engaged in embryo research will behave so badly, provoking such a public response, that legislators are forced in effect to close down the whole field?[1]

Permitting but Limiting Research

One would think that the opponents of embryo research, if they cannot win a ban, would prefer regulation that sharply limits the research rather than the status quo, which many around the world characterize as "the wild west" of American science. Rigorous regulation, which is what is being proposed here, would surely result in fewer embryos being created and destroyed than would occur without regulation. To receive permission to work with embryos, researchers would have to persuade a panel of scientific experts, ethicists, religious scholars, and others that the research can be done only by using human embryos, and only by using embryos created by the means proposed (or using donated embryos as a first choice), and with no fewer than the number proposed. Researchers would not only have to demonstrate their competence, but also show the merit of their research in advancing basic science or medical benefit. The regulatory process would reject many research proposals and limit others. Short of a ban, why is this not the preferred route for those troubled by embryo research?

It is easy, of course, to see why this is the preferred option for those of us who wish to permit limited research. Not only does it achieve what is most important—permitting but limiting research—but it also has the benefit of contributing to an emerging international consensus on embryo research. The United Kingdom and, more recently, the nation of Singapore, small but a key player in this field, have taken positions favoring limited and regulated research. The advantage found in having the major research nations take similar policies is three-fold. First, it reduces any temptation felt by scientists and corporations to relocate where regulation is limited or nonexistent. Second, it is an encouragement to other nations, which may not have the internal moral pressures but wish to be part of the global community, to take similar positions so as to maintain their place of respect among the nations. Third, international agreement contributes to the global seriousness with which the ban is regarded and thus to the likelihood that it will remain in place for a significant period of time. By contrast, winning support for a more-restrictive policy than one's international neighbors, or for a moratorium set to expire, will create disrespect for all restraints and nourish the hope of some that, one by one, all bans will fall away.

Furthermore, precisely by imposing a serious burden of regulation and limitation, such a policy expresses at least part of what we mean by "respect" for the embryo. Such respect, we believe, is limited and contingent on the actual state of the embryo and therefore not absolute. We hear too often the complaint made by critics of all embryo research that, when they hear about respect for embryos in research, they do not understand what is being said. "How can one respect an embryo and destroy it?" they ask.

Respect for the embryo is public and behavioral, not primarily private and attitudinal. No one can police the attitudes of researchers or of the public. We will never know whether they regard these tiny clusters of cells with what might be called respect or reverence or special value, or whether they experience awe at their creation and grief at their destruction. When as part of our position we demand that embryos be treated with respect, we do not imagine regulating thought but regulating research and holding it accountable to the highest standards of scientific and public responsibility. This shows precisely the limited respect we affirm. If we did not respect the embryo, we would not want to regulate research. If we respected the embryo absolutely as the equal of a person, we would ban research. Limited or contingent respect translates into a public policy of limited use. A globally coherent set of regulatory boards monitoring and limiting embryo research would be a powerful expression of universal respect for the human embryo.

To this, the critics of research argue, "This respect is allegedly demonstrated by limiting such research—and therefore limiting the numbers of embryos that may be created, used, and destroyed—to only the most serious purposes: namely, scientific investigations that hold out the potential for curing diseases or relieving suffering. But this self-limitation shows only that our purposes are steadfastly high-minded; it does not show that the *means* of pursuing these purposes are *respectful of the cloned embryos* that are necessarily violated, exploited, and destroyed in the process. To the contrary, a true respect for a being would nurture and encourage it toward its own flourishing."[2]

Let us grant that "true" or absolute respect demands a ban on research, just as a position of no respect requires no ban. Accordingly, the limited degree of respect for which we are arguing requires a policy of limiting research. The limits are the measure of respect. That the limits we propose are not absolute should not surprise the critics of research or leave them puzzled, as they sometimes claim to be. What other research policy and what other outward or institutionalized forms of respect might possibly correspond to a view that the embryo is not the moral equal of a baby, and not nothing, but something in between? Relative or limited respect requires rigorously limited use, not less but surely not more.

In fact, is it not more accurate here to say that those who insist they will either have their ban or no regulation at all are in the end showing the greatest disrespect to the embryo? Despite their intentions, which of course are otherwise, are they not offering themselves as the necessary political factor in creating a situation that imposes no limits? Their refusal to compromise by agreeing to limits or to regulated research means that they lend their unintended support to the unrestrained destruction of what they claim to hold dear.

Of course, the opponents of research will protest at this point and say that, if they agree to limited and regulated embryo research, they are in fact accepting a policy and probably a law that permits and to some extent thereby "teaches" that embryo research and embryo destruction are morally acceptable. And, even more strongly, they will protest that any policy that permits creating and using cloned embryos but prohibits reproductive cloning will thereby *require* the destruction of cloned embryos.

There may in the end be no attainable position of conscience for our friends who oppose embryo research. If they cannot win a ban, can they compromise with what they see as evil if their compromise limits what they oppose?

Notes

1. The first of these scenarios is the more likely, I think, but as one biotechnology research director once said to me, "We don't want to have happen to us what happened to nuclear power."

2. President's Council on Bioethics, "Human Cloning and Human Dignity: An Ethical Inquiry" (July 2002): 31 (available online at www.bioethics.gov/reports/ [last accessed April 22, 2003]).

SEVEN

To Be Willing to Kill What for All One Knows Is a Person Is to be Willing to Kill a Person

ROBERT SONG

A rguments about the morality of research on human embryonic stem cells have centered on a number of recurrent themes, among them the moral status of the embryonic stem cells themselves, the nature of the consent given by those who donate embryos for research, the risks associated with potential clinical applications, the propriety of public funding for this research, the dangers of the commodification of human life, the just distribution of the benefits of the research, and the questionably necessary use of embryonic stem cells if adult stem cells are able to achieve the same results. Beyond doubt, however, the most controversial issue has been that of the moral status of the embryo from which the stem cells are taken.[1] Because the extraction of stem cells from the inner cell mass at the blastocyst stage leads to the destruction of the embryo from which they are taken, the question of the ontological status of the embryo—whether it should be regarded as what I shall call, for the sake of argument, a "person"—is critical.

Of course, this is only likely to be the decisive moral concern for those who take the view that, from the time of fertilization, embryos should be given the same protection from lethal harm as that afforded to children or adults. But even those on the other side, who reject this view, cannot entirely neglect the issue, for any answer to the question of the morality of embryonic stem cell research will incorporate an implicit account of the status of the embryo. And that account, if it denies personhood to the embryo, will be required to determine, among other things, whether the embryo should be treated with respect and, if so, what practical difference such respect might make: in particular, it will need to clarify whether showing respect to an embryo is compatible with destroying it.

For these reasons, the question of the ontology of the early embryo remains crucial, and not only for those who believe that embryos should be treated as if they are persons. This is especially important to remember at a time when siren voices assure us that the matter has been "settled" or "resolved," so we are free to move onto other things. It was only proper therefore that the House of Lords Select Committee on Stem Cell Research should address this issue in its report on the issues raised by human cloning and stem cell research. This was of particular significance in the British context, because, for the previous decade and more, the matter had been regarded by official bodies as settled under the terms of the Human Fertilisation and Embryology Act 1990.[2] That statute, drawing on the recommendations made in 1984 by the government-appointed Warnock Committee, enshrined the view that the early embryo until fourteen days after fertilization (about the time of the appearance of the primitive streak) was entitled to a special status, albeit not one that gave it absolute protection. The Select Committee, however, rightly aware of the question's centrality to the ethics of stem cell research, devoted a chapter of its report to revisiting the matter. That the noble Lords felt obliged to do so, despite the embryo's status having previously been settled in law, is arguably evidence of some continuing willingness to attend to fundamental moral questions in the British public debate.

Regrettably, however, the committee's treatment of the issue was rather less satisfactory. In this chapter, I will focus on one kind of argument that it considered and leave analysis of its other claims aside. The argument I will examine, which the committee describes in terms of whether the embryo should be given the "benefit of the doubt," is one whose significance I shall maintain has been misunderstood by both its advocates and its critics.[3] Once it is correctly understood, it significantly restructures the nature of the debate and indeed imposes requirements on the arguments against the personhood of the embryo that are considerably stiffer than is usually recognized.

Persons, Doubts, and Benefits

Advocates who invoke the benefit of the doubt usually introduce the argument as a kind of tiebreaker, as a way of reaching a solution if the scores are level. If all the substantive arguments (over twinning, the notion of personhood as developmental, the relevance of the capacity for consciousness, and so on) have failed to produce a decisive conclusion one way or the other, the embryo should be given the benefit of the doubt. Indeed, the special habitat of the argument seems to be at the end of lists of reasons for attributing personhood to the embryo, where it is pressed into service in order to clinch a case that the earlier arguments may not have settled. The implicit model behind the appeal to the benefit of the doubt is of a balance of probabilities, where the evenly balanced scales will be tipped in favor of the embryo once this argument is added to the pan.

Critics of the argument often also use an unspoken picture of a pair of scales. As an example of this, consider the Select Committee's observations on the subject: "Burden of proof arguments are notoriously hard to resolve. If there were no morally serious reasons for undertaking research, then the mere possibility that the early embryo is a person would be sufficient reason not to do such research. However, if there are morally weighty reasons for doing such research a decision must be reached on the basis of arguments that fall short of proof."[4] They then note that therapies for serious diseases count as morally weighty reasons and that the idea of respect for persons can be invoked on that side of the argument as well. Here also items are being balanced against each other, the "morally weighty" reasons for undertaking research evidently being deemed sufficient to outweigh the "mere possibility" that the early embryo is a person.

It is not entirely easy to reconstruct these brief remarks in the report, but its line of reasoning appears to turn on two claims. The first seems to be that, because burden-of-proof arguments are inconclusive—though the reasons for this are unspecified—we must resort to a balance of probabilities. The second is that, in weighing the different reasons in this balance of probabilities, the mere possibility of the embryo being a person acts as a kind of reducing factor, such that the *possibility* of killing someone should be given a fraction of the weight that would be attributed to *actually* killing someone. Once that is accepted, the possibility of developing therapies for serious and common diseases then outweighs the now rather abstract notion of destroying a possible person.

Both of these claims made by the report are unfounded, for reasons that have a common cause. Moreover, for the same underlying reason, advocates who appeal to the benefit of the doubt also fail to see the force of their own argument. On both sides the force of the possibility that someone might be *killed* is lost, and the consequence is that the standard of proof required is wrongly calibrated. Both sides assume that the standard of proof required is that of a simple balance of probabilities: for advocates, the benefit of the doubt is used to tip the balance in favor of the embryo, whereas for critics the alleged problems with benefit of the doubt reasoning are used to exclude it as a consideration from the calculation of the balance of probabilities.

If what is at stake is possibly killing a person, three things immediately follow. First, a simple balance of this kind is too low a standard of proof. To see this, consider the kind of proof we would require in other situations when we are not sure if a person is present who might be killed. The supervisor of a demolition team called in to demolish a decaying factory building in which children sometimes played would not be satisfied if he were informed after a search that on the balance of probabilities no child was present. A surgical team trying to resuscitate a patient whose cardiac arrest during surgery left it unclear whether she was dead would not cease from their efforts because on a balance of probabilities she probably was dead. In each case, what would be required would be something like proof beyond reasonable doubt. Similarly, in the case of destructive research on embryos, the standard of proof required is much higher than a mere balance of probabilities: it must be shown beyond reasonable doubt (or something like this) that the embryo is not a person.

Second, in addition to there being the requirement of a heightened standard of proof, the burden of proof also falls on one side, namely, on those who would deny that there is a person present. In each of the two examples just given, the onus is on those who would deny that there is a person present to demonstrate their case. This also applies in the case of research using embryos. Of course, there are morally weighty reasons for wishing to undertake such research, notably the hope of treatments for painful and debilitating illnesses; and given the enormous benefits that allegedly could be gained from it, the temptation is naturally great to want to put the burden of proof on its opponents. Nevertheless, the burden of proof still falls on those who would deny that the embryo is a person. The reason for this is that the embryo has possibly so much more at stake, namely, its life. The value of life may not be put in a balance against the value of developing therapies for serious diseases, because life is protected by the prohibition against killing, a negative prohibition that is always binding, and it cannot be set in a balance against or outweighed by any set of positive goods, however morally desirable they may be. When therefore the Select Committee suggests that the idea of respect for persons includes respect for their health and not just respect for their (possible) life, it attempts a doctrine of equivalence that is morally untenable.

This point turns on a third, crucial consideration. The fact that the personhood of the embryo is a mere possibility cannot be used as grounds for diminishing, qualifying, or factoring down the weight to be attributed to it when considering the balance of arguments. The reason for this is that, in the words of moral theologian Germain Grisez, "to be willing to kill what for all one knows is a person is to be willing to kill a person."[5] To be willing to participate in the project of destroying an entity for whose personal status some arguments can reasonably be sustained is to be willing to participate in a project that involves killing. Rather than factoring down the moral weight to be given to embryos because of the mere possibility of their personhood, their moral weight should be factored up such that they are regarded as full persons: if, for all one knows, they are persons, they should be treated as persons. The merely possible personhood of the embryo may *seem* abstract or theoretical in comparison with the ostensibly concrete hopes for clinical treatments derived from embryonic stem cell research. But that should not be allowed to mask the true nature of the intention involved in embryo destruction.

Two clarifications of this argument must be made. First, although the proof required is of the order of proof beyond reasonable doubt, it is important to recognize that this is not proof beyond any doubt at all. To say that *for all one knows* an embryo is a person is not to concede that any remote argument, however implausible, is sufficient to require one to treat an embryo as if it is a person. Indeed, to claim that there must be no doubt at all, that it must be absolutely certain that the embryo is not a person before one could conduct research on it, would require a level of certainty that is arguably not even in principle attainable by human beings. Moreover, it would have some bizarre implications. To see this, consider the question whether scientists may carry out lethal research on animals. With regard to apes and other higher primates, there is at least some case (though I do not present the case here) for thinking that they are endowed with sufficient capacities to engender a doubt whether such research on them is justified: on this view, it is not proven beyond doubt that they are not worthy of protection. But if one were to accept that research on apes should be prohibited because we may harbor some uncertainty about their status, why not extend this prohibition to research on dogs? And if dogs, why not rabbits, mice, flies, worms, single-celled bacteria? That is, if absolute certainty beyond any doubt at all is required, perhaps even *Drosophila melanogaster* and *Caenorhabditis elegans* should be set free from the laboratories.

On the other hand, if one believes that the fruit fly and nematode worm may justifiably be experimented on, it is not because no doubt *at all* could be raised about their status (think of the quandaries that might face a Jain biologist), but because one is satisfied beyond *reasonable* doubt that they do not have a status that should protect them from lethal harm and that any substantive arguments for obligations toward them are exceptionally improbable, and therefore may be discounted. That is, doubts must be reasonable, even if it is possible life that is at stake. The alternative, requiring obligations toward life to be upheld even in cases of exceptional unlikelihood, would, as Lisa Sowle Cahill puts it, "require all suburbanites parked in locked garages to check for derelicts under their cars before they leave for work in the morning; and all parents to have every jar of baby food chemically investigated immediately prior to serving."[6]

This shows that the substantive arguments concerning the status of the embryo are not irrelevant. Recognizing the proper standard of proof required in relation to the status of the embryo is not a means of trumping the discussions about embryonic twinning and recombination, the developmental nature of personhood, and so on. Rather, the role of these substantive arguments remains: on the one side, the aim is to demonstrate that beyond reasonable doubt the embryo is not a person; on the other, to show that reasonable doubt does obtain.[7]

The second clarification is that this argument, which claims that the appropriate standard is proof beyond reasonable doubt, should not be confused with the "precautionary principle." This principle, which is widely discussed in relation to environmental planning and other public policy decisions, is invoked with a view to providing tighter safeguards against potentially bad consequences than would be obtained through conventional risk-benefit or cost-benefit analyses. Because the possible adverse consequences of, say, building a nuclear reactor or planting genetically modified crops are so severe, the principle maintains, we should not act unless we can be sure that no harm will be done.

The two approaches do of course bear a superficial similarity: the one presses for a standard of proof beyond reasonable doubt instead of proof on a balance of probabilities, and the other invokes the precautionary principle of not taking action unless no harm will be done in preference to a conventional cost-benefit analysis. This similarity is often thought to license use of the latter approach to model the former. An example of this might be a comparison of the embryo research case with a hypothetical decision whether to build a road transport system. Those who defend the analogy claim that refusing to research on embryos because of the possibility that embryonic persons might be killed would be like refusing to have a road system because of the possibility that people might be killed. Life involves risk, they urge: without being willing to undergo risk, one will never achieve anything. Moreover, risks have to be quantified, and this involves attributing values to the lives of those who will die. On an ordinary cost-benefit analysis, the expectation that people will be killed is outweighed by the prospective benefits brought by a road system. By contrast, the adoption of a precautionary principle would be inappropriate, inasmuch as it would likely be a "recipe for stasis."[8] By analogy, holding up scientific and medical research because of concerns about proving beyond reasonable doubt the nonpersonhood of the embryo is a way of ensuring that important medical advances will be significantly and unnecessarily hindered.

The analogy, however, does not hold. Aside from its ready empirical assumption that embryonic stem cell research is a necessary means to the desired therapeutic end, it also factors down the deaths of possible embryo persons, failing to recognize that to be willing to kill what for all one knows is a person is to be willing to kill a person, in the way we have already discussed. Perhaps most importantly, it fails to notice the different kind of logic each approach has. The precautionary principle is set within a consequentialist matrix, in which different outcomes are each assigned a value and probabilities are attached to their occurring. Rather than a simple net utility being the criterion, as would be the case in a straightforward cost-benefit analysis, the precautionary principle proposes that, even if a simple overall calculus on balance favored a project, it should be rejected if the disutility of the bad outcomes (however small their probability) were sufficiently great. Equally, rebuttal of the precautionary principle is likely to appeal to consequences, typically taking the form of showing that its adoption would lead to worse outcomes than adopting a standard cost-benefit approach.

The balance of probabilities that I have discussed in relation to the morality of embryo research has a different set of concerns. Here it is not the consequences of different actions that are being weighed against each other, but rather the quality of different arguments. Although superficially it could seem as if a utilitarian calculus lay behind the picture of the weighing scales, the issue is of discerning how much intellectual weight to give to different moral arguments. The beyond-reasonable-doubt standard of proof, together with its corollaries I discussed above, is an effort to determine the level of cogency arguments on each side must possess if they are to carry the day. Equally, rebutting it requires moral argument, not just a demonstration of the (allegedly) bad consequences of adopting it.

It is also worth noting that, even if one did wish to press the analogy, there is a substantial moral difference between the two cases. To return to the example of the road system, the deaths of road users are at no point directly intended or desired by the planners. Moreover, in no sense can their deaths be said to be necessary to the good functioning of the roads. It would be quite conceivable that one could have a road system in which no one ever died, and indeed engineers go to (greater or lesser) lengths to try to achieve this. In the case of embryo research, by contrast, destroying embryos is the necessary and unavoidable means to the end of obtaining stem cells or doing embryo research. There is no "risk" that they will die. Rather, their deaths are an intrinsic part of the process. Or at least, if their deaths are avoidable, then the objection to embryo research on the grounds of the possible personhood of the embryo falls! The proper analogy would be with designing a road transport system in which an indefinite number of people would be deliberately and unavoidably killed as an intrinsic part of the process of building and operating it.

As should be clear, none of the above considerations determines whether embryos should be treated as if they are persons. The substantive arguments in favor of embryo research may not be able to demonstrate embryonic nonpersonhood beyond reasonable doubt, and the substantive arguments against it may not be able to show that their scruples on behalf of embryos are reasonable. I cannot review here the range of arguments deployed on either side, beyond making some preliminary comments.

First, it is my conviction that the arguments in favor of the personhood of the early embryo certainly are strong enough to sustain a reasonable doubt whether embryos may ever be subjected to lethal research. Indeed, there are good grounds for believing that they are at least as cogent as those favoring a later start for personhood than fertilization, if not more so.[9]

Second, the public determination of whether the case is proven beyond reasonable doubt must make use of some conception of public reasoning.[10] This should not be regarded as something that by definition excludes religious convictions from the public realm. Public reason is not a matter of abstract appeals to putative canons of "full rationality" as constructed by secular norms, but instead the embodied disputation of historical communities whose commitments sometimes overlap, sometimes diverge. Some arguments that are made from within particular traditions may be readily accessible and appealing to those outside of those traditions, whereas others are only likely to be attractive to those who share the same fundamental vision of the good. What is regarded as beyond reasonable doubt in relation to embryo research is therefore inevitably likely to be contested, but at all events those whose judgments of the matter are informed by religious commitments may not be dismissed as speaking merely "private" languages of no public relevance. Of course, for legal and practical purposes, the issue will need to be finally settled by the procedures a political society lays down for itself, and it may be that conscientious citizens find themselves in fundamental moral opposition to provisions made by the law. In such circumstances, they will do well to recall the traditional natural law declaration that an unjust law is not a law and does not of itself have the power of binding the conscience.

Acknowledgments

This chapter grows out of presentations made to the Colloquy on the Religious and Moral Implications of Embryonic Stem Cell Research, held at Garrett-Evangelical Theological Seminary, Evanston, Illinois, in October 2001, and the House of Lords Select Committee on Stem Cell Research, St. John's College, Durham, in November 2001.

Notes

1. On the moral issues surrounding embryonic stem cell research, see in general Suzanne Holland, Karen Lebacqz, and Laurie Zoloth, eds., *The Human Embryonic Stem Cell Debate: Science, Ethics and Public Policy* (Cambridge, Mass.: MIT Press, 2001), though note that this book does little to analyze the significance of recent developments in adult and primitive nonembryonic stem cell research.

2. House of Lords Select Committee on Stem Cell Research, *Report from the Select Committee,* HL 83 (London: HMSO, 2002) (available at www.publications.parliament. uk/pa/ld/ldstem.htm) [accessed 10 January 2003]. The committee was set up under the terms of the Human Fertilisation and Embryology (Research Purposes) Regulations 2001. These regulations extended the Human Fertilisation and Embryology Act 1990, the principal U.K. legislation related to infertility treatment and research, so as to permit embryonic stem cell research. In an effort to address the moral concerns raised during the House of Lords debate on the bill, the regulations also required that a committee be established to consider and report on the issues raised by human cloning and stem cell research. That

the committee was set up to consider the morality of the legislation *after* the legislation had been passed raised unavoidable questions about its credibility.

3. The argument is discussed in paragraphs 4.15–17 of the report.

4. Ibid., paragraph 4.16.

5. Germain Grisez, *The Way of the Lord Jesus*, vol. 2: *Living a Christian Life* (Quincy, Ill.: Franciscan Press, 1993), 497.

6. Lisa Sowle Cahill, "The Embryo and the Fetus: New Moral Contexts," *Theological Studies* 54 (1993): 124–42, at 131.

7. The same considerations in principle apply in the case of animals. Although this chapter does not attend to these questions, we should note (1) the implications of the beyond-reasonable-doubt principle may end up encompassing a wider range of nonhuman animals than we may initially find comfortable; (2) the fact that we may be morally required to extend protection beyond the human species is not as such an argument for denying that protection to those entities that are unquestionably of the human species, even if they are not children or full-grown adults.

8. Julian Morris, ed., *Rethinking Risk and the Precautionary Principle* (Oxford: Butterworth-Heinemann, 2000), viii.

9. See further my treatment of stem cell research and the moral status of the embryo in *Human Genetics: Fabricating the Future* (Cleveland: Pilgrim Press, 2002), 30–40. For a recent statement to which I am sympathetic, see David Jones, *Cloning and Stem Cell Research* (London: Linacre Centre, 2001); available at www.linacre.org/stemcell.html [accessed 10 January 2003]. See also the literature cited there.

10. On public reason in a pluralist society, see my *Christianity and Liberal Society* (Oxford: Clarendon Press, 1997), 213–33.

PART THREE

Research

EIGHT

A Plea for Beneficence: Reframing the Embryo Debate

TED PETERS AND GAYMON BENNETT

The birth of Dolly the sheep in 1997 inspired a rare phenomenon: near moral unanimity. Since that fateful February day, virtually everyone on the planet has been opposed to bringing children into the world through reproductive cloning. In June and July 2002, two high-level government reports, one in Singapore and the other in the United States, reiterated this shared opposition, recommending a total ban on the use of somatic cell nuclear transfer in human reproduction.[1] The bans have met almost no resistance. Whether the explanation is found in a shared worldwide ethical sensibility or in the lack of imagined ways to turn a profit from reproductive cloning, something close to unanimity reigns.[2] Despite the actions of renegade off-shore cloners, theological ethicists have found influencing public policy to be easy. In such a situation, ethical arguments tend not to be carefully examined, and rhetoric is rarely scrutinized. What may become public policy in many countries will be established on consensus, to be sure; yet, when in later years philosophers look back for fundamental premises, they may not find a solid foundation.

By contrast, the stem cell debate—entailing the question of whether cloning should be used for research—continues to be vigorous, spirited, and sometimes acrimonious. Venture capitalists with eyes fixed on potential big profits mix with laboratory scientists, theological ethicists, secular ethicists, and public policy makers. The public square is riddled by crossfire from ethical guerrillas, each faction contending for the disputed laboratory territory.

The stem cell itself is not the turf to be won; rather, it is the moral status of the embryo from which the stem cell is derived. The public battle requires that each faction return frequently to its philosophical armory to load up and strengthen its position in combat. In the case of theological ethics, theologians must return again and again to fundamental convictions about God's intention for human nature and destiny.

Though still exchanging shots, the factions have reached a stalemate, neither retreating nor advancing. This is due in large part to a combination of ideological entrenchment and the incommensurability of differing principles; however, it is also due to the caliber of ammunition being used in the exchange. In the rush to defend and advance, scientists, philosophers, and theologians alike have often not reached deep enough into the resources of their respective traditions. The result has been that the weighty ethical payload of moral arguments has been launched from less than stable foundations. Moral advances are weakened by incomplete ethical reflection.

In the present chapter, we will examine a crucial cause of this ethical incompleteness: the failure of beneficence to count substantively in ethical deliberation assessing the moral status of the embryo. We will outline this failure by examining the conclusions and supporting arguments of the two government reports from nearly opposite sides of the planet, the Singapore Bioethics Advisory Committee (the BAC) and the American President's Council on Bioethics (the Kass council). We will show how both reports found it easy to recommend government bans on reproductive cloning, and how that ease can belie a negative disposition toward moral responsibility. We will show further how much more difficult the respective investigations found the issue of cloning for research, with its implications for stem cell derivation and how this difficulty results in ambivalence. Although the Singapore report recommends support for stem cell research, ambivalence is reflected in its preference list for sources of research embryos. Although the American report includes a majority recommendation for a four-year moratorium on cloning for use in stem cell research, it includes a minority recommendation to support such research.

This nearly irresolvable situation in public policy compels church leaders to reexamine theological commitments, to reconsider what is foundational and what might be applicable or helpful. This reexamination begins with theological anthropology. It is our contention that Christian anthropology is characterized by (1) eschatological destiny, (2) the morally compelling value of the human person, or what is more commonly articulated as the affirmation of human dignity, and (3) the fundamental (meaning both primordial and universal) imperative of *agape* or neighbor love. This definition suggests to us that beneficence should play a basic role in bioethics.

Our support of beneficence will not resolve the stem cell debate to everyone's satisfaction. Our arguments are neither airtight, nor, for that matter, complete. They are in process, our articulation inspired by a perceived lack in the current debate. Yet, we have something to offer to theologians and other church leaders involved in the public policy conversation. Our immediate contention is that the public policy debate would be healthier if all commentators would allow beneficence to count more significantly in their ethical calculus.[3] We would like to see the potential leap forward in human health and well-being promised by stem cell research play a role (at minimum) equal to that of nonmaleficence—that is, equal to a guarding against future harms and the protection of the embryo. Responsibility cast in positive terms inspires a move beyond the status quo of human suffering. Though the prevention of harm is crucial, proscriptions against crossing moral bright lines should be balanced by prescriptions for active stewarding of resources to improve human life.

Our more long-range contention is that theologians should be reminded that definitions of what makes us human rely less on our origin and more on our destiny, less on our creation and more on our new creation. In other words, what is significant about who we are now is not found in our genetic past, but in God's future—a resurrected future where suffering is transformed and life is had to the fullest.

Eschatology, Dignity, and Beneficence

The stem cell and cloning debates reveal inconsistencies in contemporary Christian anthropology and its application to bioethics. Beneficence often fails to function substantively in theological assessments of the moral status of the embryo and, hence, in the stem cell and cloning debates. We are persuaded that this has less to do with ignorance or ill will and more to do with poorly developed anthropology. Theological contributions to public debate are frustrated by dissonant interpretations of what constitutes ethical responsibility and morally protectable human life.

A curious phenomenon pervades virtually all human cultures and traditions. When seeking identity and meaningfulness, our minds tend to gravitate toward the past, toward origins. Whatever the reason for this phenomenon, we find a coincidence of the questions "Who am I?" and "Where did I come from?" In the stem cell debate, these anthropological questions become "When did life begin?" and "How is each person's unique human potential established?" and "What does that establishment tell me about how humans should be treated?" The unexamined assumption in this line of questioning is that, once we have located the ontogenesis or beginning, we will have located the defining source of our moral selfhood. In other words, if we discover just where it is that we come from, we will be compelled in the ethical direction we ought to be moving.

The Roman Catholic Church, with its modern history of commentary on the status of the embryo, was well positioned to be the first to define the theological agenda for the stem cell debate. Pope John Paul II and the Congregation for the Doctrine of the Faith had already, in 1987, provided answers to the question of moral ontogenesis.[4] In *Donum Vitae* the Vatican reiterates a previously articulated conclusion: that protectable human life begins at conception. *Donum Vitae,* however, takes what was formerly a philosophical/theological conclusion and spells it out in semiscientific terms. The recipe for personhood requires three ingredients: sperm, egg, and soul. At conception, when the sperm and egg join, God creates and imparts an immortal soul. The united gametes and soul constitute a new human individual endowed with dignity and worthy of the respect and protection due any adult or child. Of course, the conceptus is not at this early stage in itself a human person. It is, however, a human person in potential. Its genetic code is new, neither its mother's nor father's alone. It can become this person and no other.

This genomic novelty carries anthropological and ethical weight for the Vatican. It designates at what point we should apply the principle of inviolability, a universal marker of a morally protectable person. Evangelical Protestants, whose traditions may not have traveled the same arduous course of ethical deliberation, tend to respond intuitively to the Roman Catholic arguments. They affirm that the Vatican has it right.

The conclusions of other early commentators on embryo research have also helped set the moral agenda of the stem cell debate. Though with less appeal to metaphysics, these too answered the question of moral origins. Some have argued that morally protectable human dignity begins at fourteen days. This fourteen-day rule argues that, prior to the appearance of the primitive streak, a precursor to the central nervous system, and adherence to the uterine wall, the embryo is not truly individuated. Prior to fourteen days, the embryo can still become twins. Thus, it is not until fourteen days that we have the clear appearance of the individual human life.

Much like the Vatican, the fourteen-day rule looks for the origins of personhood in individuation. Though the appeal is not made to genetic uniqueness, the fourteen-day rule seems to concur that characteristics of respect and inviolability are meaningless until we have an individual person to whom we can apply those characteristics.

We find it significant that both an appeal to genetic uniqueness and the fourteen-day rule exemplify archonic reasoning. Archonic reasoning privileges the point of origin. It assumes that the essence of a thing is found in its beginnings. Archonism looks to the past for metaphysical or physical grounding of moral authority. The essence of the origin, it is presumed, will serve as ethical edict for the present situation.

The Greek word *arche* means both beginning and governance. The way in which a thing begins decrees or governs the direction in which it ought to continue. Contemporary genetic research seems to provide a new means of grounding archonic reasoning. By researching the biological "blueprint" for the beginnings of human life, we should be able to fashion moral prescriptions directing our human future. Both the appeal to genetic novelty and the fourteen-day rule appear to draw out of biology the moral authority of archonism.

We have suggested that theological anthropology needs to be reexamined. This reappraisal begins with the question, "Should archonic reasoning be privileged by Christian theologians?" Our answer is flatly, "No." What is distinctive about Christian anthropology is that it is oriented toward the future, a transformed and just future. The Christian understanding of the human person, counterintuitively, begins not in creation, with who we are, but in redemption, with who we are intended to be.

For the Christian, the identity, value, and meaningfulness of the human person are inextricably bound up in Jesus of Nazareth. Jesus announces and proleptically realizes God's eschatological destiny for creation. That announcement and realization reveals God's active, self-giving, and redemptive love and in doing so reveals the truth of human identity. The character of God's love for creation testifies to the true nature of who we are. The Kingdom of God, according to Jesus, is characterized by sight for the blind, functioning limbs for the lame, healing for those with leprosy, hearing for the deaf, new life for the dead, and good news for the poor (Luke 7:22–23). Jesus locates our fundamental identity not in the archonic roots of injustice, but in God's graceful future, a future which responds to human suffering, promising healing and offering the flourishing of life.

What anthropological generalizations can be drawn here? Jesus' vision of God's love suggests that who we are is inextricably tied up in who we are becoming, who we will be. Who we will be, in turn, is inextricably tied up in who the Easter Christ is—that is, we will realize who we truly are in the resurrection. In sum, what is most true about us is not revealed in our genetic origins but in the epigenetic history of God's relationship to each person in Christ. Eschatologically, we will become one with Christ and like Christ and live in Christ.

The vision of God's eschatological destiny for creation is morally compelling. It reveals not only the truth of human identity, but also the significance of human value and the imperative of neighbor love. God's love confers dignity on creatures. That conferring testifies to the way in which the human person ought to be valued and related to.

Human dignity seems to imply individuality, even radical independence. After all, our concept of dignity as formulated by Immanuel Kant makes it clear that we treat a person—an individual person—as an end and not merely as a means.[5] Yet the individuality of dignity has a relational dimension to it. It is in the relationship, wherein a person experiences being treated by someone else as an end and not a means; once dignity has been conferred by someone else, one's own internal sense of dignity arises. Dignity is first conferred, and then it is claimed. Dignity is conferred on individuals, but it is established in relationship.

For the Christian, God's relationship to creation, described and exemplified by Jesus, represents the conferring of dignity par excellence. In the Gospel of Luke (6:27–36), Jesus' understanding of God's relationship to human persons is described in this way: Jesus proclaims that we should love persons not as we think they deserve to be loved, but indiscriminately, as God loves them. God, Jesus reports, loves the good and wicked alike. Again, human value is revealed not in an archonic assessment of human worth—where people have come from—but according to the human person's future as beloved, completed and redeemed by God. Human dignity is measured by God's perfect and perfecting love.

A Christian anthropology that begins with Jesus is morally compelling in a second way. Danish philosopher Knud Løgstrup points out that Jesus' proclamation is concerned with the individual's relationship to the neighbor.[6] According to Løgstrup, this concern can be concisely described: the individual's relationship with God is determined at the point of the individual's relationship to the human neighbor. Moreover, it is precisely at the point where God determines his relationship to me that he cares for the other person. God's eschatological love for the other person is bound up in my relationship to that person. Face to face with the human other, I am confronted with a tremendous obligation—to participate in God's redemption of the world through what Martin Luther refers to as "neighbor-love."

Jesus articulates this primordial obligation in the parable of the Good Samaritan. When asked what it takes to participate in the Kingdom of God, Jesus answers, Love God and love your neighbor. Jesus' interrogator pushes the question: what does that love look like? Jesus replies with a story. The Samaritan (born of the wrong nation, subscribing to the wrong theology) single-mindedly purses one goal, to bring healing to someone suffering and in need. This is an active, aggressive form of love, one that takes initiative and acts creatively. In short, when asked what is most significant about human existence Jesus points to a commandment, an imperative to participate in God's healing of the world through the love of one's neighbor.

Christian anthropology does not begin with Adam (Genesis 1:26–29; 2:7), but with Jesus Christ (Romans 5). The problem with archonic anthropology when pursued by Christian theologians is that it looks to Adam rather than Christ, to creation without redemption. Proleptically, humans participate in the grace of God's eschatological destiny. Ethically speaking, grace appears to reorder reason. God's love identifies us with the future truth of who we are becoming, not with the merits of our genetic inheritance. Taking this vision of human dignity as our moral norm, we find ourselves responsible not only for what we did or willed, for our own faults and misfortunes. But, with Jesus, we find ourselves called to account for that which we may not have willed or done: the faults, misfortunes, and suffering of others.

In the end, it is not enough for Christian anthropology merely to inspire an ethic of proportionality, fairness, just deserts, or distributive equality, even if, relatively speaking, an ethic of equality lends itself well to public policy recommendations in a democratic context. Rather, Christian anthropology should inspire the pursuit of the other person's well-being toward the end of that person having what Jesus referred to as life, and having it to its fullest (John 10:10). Christian anthropology depicts the truth of human ethics as a going out of one's way for the healing and wholeness of one's most intimate friend, one's most feared enemy, and even for the faceless stranger.

The bioethical correlative of this active and determined neighbor-love is beneficence. The degree to which bioethical reflection fails to treat beneficence as a substantive factor in its moral calculus determines the degree to which it fails to draw on distinctively Christian resources.

The Singapore BAC

In June 2002, the BAC, chaired by Professor Lim Pin, submitted its report to Deputy Prime Minister Tony Tan. The report describes its central task in terms of ethical balancing. The gravity of questions concerning the moral status of the embryo is weighed against the need to harness potential medical benefits. This task is framed according to two guiding principles. When exploiting the benefits of science and technology, the pursued ends must be (1) just and (2) sustainable.[7]

The BAC clearly saw the potential benefits of embryonic stem cell research and promotes investment in this area. The promotion, however, is wed to substantial caveat. Note the language in Recommendation 3: "Research involving the derivation and use of ES [embryonic stem] cells is permissible only where there is strong scientific merit in, and potential medical benefit from, such research."[8] This would seem to go without saying. Without potential benefit, why pursue any course of medical research? The caveats become increasingly interesting as the BAC constructs a hierarchy of preferred sources for human embryonic stem (hES) cell derivation. According to Recommendation 4, "Where permitted, ES cells should be drawn from sources in the following order: (1) existing ES cell lines, originating from ES cells derived from embryos less than 14 days old; and (2) surplus human embryos created for fertility treatment less than 14 days old."[9] But could a scientist create a fresh embryo to obtain hES cells as will probably be needed if stem cell research goes to therapy? Only after these first two options would be exhausted.

Recommendation 5 expands the hierarchy, offering a third option, namely, the controversial creation of fresh embryos for research purposes: "The creation of human embryos specifically for research can be justified only where (1) there is strong merit in, and potential medical benefit from, such research; (2) no acceptable alternative exists, and (3) on a highly selective, case-by-case basis, with specific approval from the proposed statutory body."[10]

With consistent emphasis on both the potential benefits of stem cell research and the need for ethical caution concerning the status of the embryo, ambivalence seems to be at work. On the one hand, the Singapore BAC is convinced that research on stem cells, even if it involves therapeutic cloning, should go forward. Further, the assumption is made here that, prior to fourteen days, when the embryo adheres to the uterine wall and the primitive streak appears, we do not have a morally protectable human being—that is, no moral proscriptions deny the blastocyst to researchers. On the other hand, the Singapore BAC grants a degree of respect to the conceptus; it is reluctant to allow embryos at the blastocyst stage to be treated without any moral regard. The BAC introduces a calculus, namely, a preferential list of approvable derivations ranked according to levels of respect shown to the early embryo. The ambivalence at work here is one that we all feel, but it is difficult to move ethical deliberation forward when caught between competing moral obligations. The task of ethicists in this situation is to help us work through the ambivalence. Establishing weight-bearing foundations, ethicists need to construct arguments capable of informing firm decisions and setting public policies.

The U.S. President's Council on Bioethics

On 9 August 2001, U.S. President George Bush addressed his nation on the controversial matter of stem cell research and the public policy debate surrounding it. In the months that followed, he appointed members to serve on the President's Council on Bioethics, directed by Leon Kass, a professor at the University of Chicago. After six months work, on 10 July 2002, Kass and appointees sent to the White House a report titled "Human Cloning and Human Dignity: An Ethical Inquiry."[11]

Concerning what it calls "cloning-to-produce-children," the U.S. report agrees with the Singapore document. The council unanimously recommends an indefinite federal ban. On what the report calls "cloning-for-biomedical-research" and its integral relationship to embryonic stem cell research, the council splits. The majority recommends a four-year moratorium, and the minority that cloning techniques be used to support stem cell research.

In the report's cover letter to President Bush, Kass cautions, "Cloning represents a turning point in human history . . . [carrying] with it a number of troubling consequences for children, family, and society."[12] It is noteworthy that this letter mentions only the troubling consequences of this historic turning point. Unacknowledged is the possibility of scientific breakthroughs; no suggestion is made that the advance of cloning technology could yield benefits to animal breeding or that cloning used for research might contribute to medicine's alleviation of human suffering.

The consideration of potential harms is crucial to responsible ethical reflection; both the majority and minority recommendations rightly grapple with the possible consequences of unexamined pursuit of science-based technology. But proscriptions against harm must be balanced by prescriptions for healing. One need not disagree with their conclusions to recognize that the majority's ethical reflection is guided almost exclusively by nonmalfeasance, a careful guarding against forecasted harm. By contrast, concern for stewarding resources to improve human well-being, or beneficence, is demoted to a secondary consideration. This demotion effectively disallows serious consideration of primary concerns related to theological anthropology as we understand it. It exemplifies the narrowing of ethics from active responsibility for healing to concern for not making matters worse.

Cloning and Babies

The council found unanimity on the one issue where everyone seems to agree: we should not use cloning to make human babies.[13] Six reasons were offered. The first is familiar cloning debate fare: safety. The council contends that cloning to produce children is unethical and recommends that it be banned by law. The Kass council attends to two previous reports, President Clinton's National Bioethics Advisory Commission, 1997, and the National Academy of Sciences, 2002. These reports oppose reproductive cloning for safety reasons. The Kass report follows suit.[14]

The five additional reasons are less familiar: (1) identity—cloned children may be expected to copy in every respect the life of the "original"; (2) manufacture—cloned children may be considered products rather than "gifts" to be treasured; (3) new eugenics—cloned children might be designed to avoid genetic defects or enhance their genetically influenced life chances; (4) troubled family relations—cloning could "confound" and "transgress" "natural boundaries" between generations, allowing fathers to be genetic twins of sons, mothers of daughters; (5) society—cloning might affect the way we look at children, introducing novel forms of intergenerational control.[15]

A notable characteristic of these five reasons is that they all depend on possible future scenarios; they worry about what might happen should reproductive cloning be practiced. This argument against cloning is an argument based on imagined deleterious effects. These arguments do not appeal to any intrinsic violations of human dignity; nor do they appeal to any identifiable theological criteria. None is based on repugnance or natural law theory or

God's will. In light of what we said earlier about the contrast between archonic and future oriented reasoning, we simply observe that on this issue the Kass council bypasses archonic assumptions. The domain of its concern is the future, in this case a speculative future.

Although we can concur with the Kass council that a ban on cloning to produce children is morally advisable at this time, we find the argumentation to be tendentious and at places superficial. Little or no medical benefits will come of reproductive uses of cloning. Moreover, those who do support reproductive cloning usually justify their views with some form of parental narcissism, that is, they seek a cloned child for selfish reasons, treating the cloned child instrumentally. The fact that the council's majority turns their moral attention almost exclusively toward potentially negative scenarios might seem unproblematic, yet it discloses a strictly negative disposition toward moral responsibility in general.

Cloning and Stem Cells

Unanimity against reproductive cloning was easy to achieve; the council, however, could not obtain unanimity on therapeutic cloning, on what it calls *cloning for biomedical research*. Like the rest of society, the council could not resolve the stem cell controversy.

Two positions within the council offer moral arguments in support of cloning for biomedical research.[16] Seven members (a minority) articulated what the report calls "position one," advocating that research proceed under strict federal regulation. Position one displays a mood of serious moral concern. The support offered does not advocate research at any cost, nor does it offer up the potential scientific gain as a moral trump card. Keeping with the tone of the entire report, they carefully acknowledge the ethical difficulties of this research while tentatively recommending that we go forward. Some of the poignant ambivalence seen with the Singapore BAC appears here as well.

Position one wrestles with four ethical difficulties: intermediate moral status, deliberate creation for use, going too far, and other moral hazards.

Intermediate Moral Status

The eye of the hurricane in public policy debate over research on hES cells has been the moral status of the early embryo. The position one minority speaks to this cautiously but clearly: "We believe there are sound moral

reasons for not regarding the embryo in its earliest stages as the moral equivalent of a human person. We believe the embryo has a developing and intermediate moral worth that commands our special respect, but that it is
morally permissible to use early-stage cloned human embryos in important
research under strict regulation."[17]

Deliberate Creation for Use

Like the Singapore BAC, the U.S. council felt it needed to address the derivation question: should we limit research to discarded frozen embryos, or
should we deliberately create fresh embryos that will be taken apart when re-
trieving hES cells? Most existing stem cell lines were derived from frozen excess embryos, although at least one was derived from a fresh embryo. It appears that fresh embryos have research advantages over frozen ones, meaning
that we can expect future pressure to produce embryos for research purposes.
The language used by the council minority instructs us here: "These embryos
would not be 'created for destruction,' but for use in the service of life and
medicine. They would be destroyed in the service of a great good, and this
should not be obscured."[18]

Going Too Far

Minority position one wants to prevent early embryos from developing so
long that they approach the fetal stage. "We approve, therefore, only of research on cloned embryos that is strictly limited to the first fourteen days of
development."[19] Minority position one within the Kass council supports the
fourteen-day rule.

Other Moral Hazards

More and more voices in the public debate can be heard registering concern
over the justice implications of gathering human eggs for scientific research,
justice concerns that focus on the health and well-being of women who donate the eggs. In addition, a slippery slope fear has arisen. Some fear that, if
we approve cloning in stem cell research, we could slide gradually toward approving reproductive cloning as well. Position one confronts these matters:
"We believe that concerns about the exploitation of women and about the
risk that cloning-for-biomedical-research could lead to cloning-to-produce-
children can be adequately addressed by appropriate rules and regulations.

These concerns need not frighten us into abandoning an important avenue of research."[20] Much like the Singapore BAC, position one recommends that the potential for future harms be guarded against by means of careful regulation. Thus qualified, position one recommends support of therapeutic cloning and related areas of research such as stem cells.

Minority "position two" within the Kass council offers similar support for cloning for biomedical research, but this position is much less timid about the moral reservations defined and dealt with above. Position two accords no special status to the early embryo. As such, it sees little reason to impede research that may revolutionize medicine. Position two argues that the cloned embryo "should be treated essentially like all other human cells."[21] In short, they do not accept the assumption that research involving cloning for biomedical research involves substantially novel moral issues, but rather that it involves concerns that accompany all human biomedical research. Position two offers categorical support for stem cell research.

Ten members of the Kass council, a majority, make the case against cloning for biomedical research. They do not recommend a total ban, but instead advocate a four-year moratorium applicable to all researchers regardless of whether federal funds are involved. The majority recommendation argues that it is morally wrong to "exploit and destroy developing human life, even for good reasons."[22] They see this research as opening doors to a morally unwise future. Moreover, they believe research on embryos is viscerally unsettling. "We find it disquieting, even somewhat ignoble, to treat what are in fact seeds of the next generation as mere raw material for satisfying the needs of our own."[23]

This argument against therapeutic cloning swings on a two-piece moral hinge. The weight-bearing piece of the hinge is the moral status of the cloned embryo. The majority rejects the claims of minority position two. They argue that the early-stage embryo is indeed quite unlike other human cells. Position two, according to the majority, "denies the continuous history of human individuals from the embryonic to fetal to infant stages of existence."[24] The majority position finds similar fault with the arguments invoked in position one, judging the concept of the intermediate status of the embryo to be unconvincing. They find invoking "special respect" for nascent human life "to have little or no operative meaning if cloned embryos may be created in bulk and used routinely with impunity."[25]

The cooperative piece on which the majority argument hinges concerns the deleterious affects resulting from a misunderstanding of the significance of potentiality. Failing to recognize the potential human life of the embryo as, de facto, a prohibition against embryonic research exhibits an ignorance of "the hazardous moral precedent that the routinized creation, use, and destruction of nascent human life would establish."[26]

What worries the Kass council majority is that we as a society will instrumentalize early human life and lose our sense of awe and respect, and that this instrumentalization could dull our social sensitivities. Cloning even for biomedical research risks crossing a "significant moral boundary. . . . Doing so would coarsen our moral sensibilities and make us a different society: one less humble toward that which we cannot fully understand, less willing to extend the boundaries of human respect outward, and more willing to transgress moral boundaries once it appears to be in our own interests to do so."[27]

While appreciating the majority's careful concern for the future well-being of society's moral sensitivity, we question the social naïveté that lends rhetorical strength to their position. Implied in their argument is that, generally speaking, society's corporate conscience is attuned to the noninstrumental value of human life. Unfortunately, this is often not the case. The ethical status quo worldwide is already quite unacceptable. We live in a society marred by a good deal of exploitation, instrumental abuse, and manipulation of human life. If cloning exacerbates these undesirable conditions society will not be different, only sadly worse.

As thoughtfully articulated and reasonable as they may be, the possible troublesome consequences enumerated by the majority are nothing more than speculative possibilities. Can we, with any degree of certainty, know that through the use of cloning a society, which does not guarantee health insurance for many of the sick children already living among us, will have its moral sensitivity to the value of developing life coarsened beyond what it already is? If not, should we invoke this troubling possibility as justification for shutting down potentially life-saving research?

This existing state of suffering and injustice thrusts on us a profound moral obligation to make things better. Implied in making things better is not letting things get worse (i.e., concerning ourselves with the prevention of future harms). The opposite does not hold true: concern for not doing further harm does not carry with it a mandate to make existing ills better.

Back to Beneficence

The leadership Leon Kass has shown in producing such a thorough piece of scholarship over a relatively short period of time is admirable. So also is his willingness to report both the majority and minority positions so that the public can see the level of difficulty at producing consensus. It is also plea-surable to think that the White House will likely be reading an eloquent ar-ticulation of wholesome values protecting the dignity of children and warn-ing society away from insensitivity toward the value of human life.

Yet, minority position one in this report has distinct merit. It stands in con-trast to much of the report in the way it frames its basic argumentation, and its attentiveness to beneficence accords well with our view that beneficence should be central to a theologically based ethic. Whether articulated as the Jewish mandate to heal or the Christian commitment to love of neighbor, theologically informed beneficence reframes bioethics. Here beneficence be-gins with the constructive vision of God's desire to heal the world. The vi-sion is basic, foundational. Hence, the first and framing question beneficence asks in the cloning debate is, Can biomedical technology be pressed into the service of healing and human well-being?

In light of injustices associated with for-profit medicine, where research dollars are usually poured into the development of treatments that offer the best return on investment, there are those that might answer "no" to the first beneficence question. These might argue that resources should be spent in meeting basic medical needs rather than pursuing therapies on the frontier of genetic science. While recognizing endemic problems with the current medical system, we choose to answer "yes." Stem cell research and cloning for research purposes can and should be pressed into the service of healing.

The model here is the Good Samaritan in Jesus' parable (Luke 10:29–37). The Samaritan pursues one goal: healing for the suffering stranger. This is an other-seeking form of love, one that takes the initiative and acts to bring about constructive change. This love defines its task according to the needs of the neighbor.

Medical science and its taxpayer support can be seen as a social form of neighbor loving, an investment on the part of the present generation for the health and welfare of the coming generation. What's more, medical research science, in its own way, contributes to God's healing work on earth. To ig-nore this divine mandate is itself an ethical concern. So many human diseases that shorten life and cause suffering could possibly find therapies through stem cell research: heart disease, cancers, organ deterioration, Alzheimer's and other brain malfunction.

Could we ask that beneficence count more in the public debate? If so, what would happen? Appeal to beneficence does not promote cloning to produce children; so living with the unanimous Kass council recommendation will be easy. In fact, theological beneficence does not necessarily require support of cloning for research, though it certainly encourages us in this direction; however, marginalizing beneficence when arguing against stem cell research, in this case against cloning for biomedical research, is lopsided. The Kass council report certainly acknowledges the potential medical benefits to which such research may lead, but this fails to function substantively in the majority argument.

Regardless of the role of the beneficence principle, there is no way to avoid facing a decisive question: when does morally protectable individual human life begin? The question invokes archonic reasoning. As such, it will significantly affect every other component to an ethical argument. Whether we date morally protectable dignity prior to the blastocyst stage or later than the blastocyst stage will determine whether we advocate hES cell research.

Keep in mind that our warrant for support of beneficence is an eschatologically informed theological anthropology. This understanding of the human person serves to answer the question behind the question of the status of the embryo, an alloyed question composed of equal parts ethics and anthropology: How ought we to understand moral responsibility for other people?

We argue that ethics should be future oriented, seeking to transform suffering into justice. A relational understanding of human dignity and the obligation to love actively and creatively underwrite this ethics. Our argument differs in form from the Vatican's appeal to genetic novelty and even to the fourteen-day rule, both of which are reasoned archonically. According to both positions, dignity is tied up in being an individual. Responsibility, here, risks being cast in strictly negative terms, as a prohibition against violating the intrinsic dignity correlative to the human individuation.

Better Safe than Sorry

We cannot, however, avoid the question, At what point during embryonic development does moral responsibility kick in? We recognize that human dignity is revealed in God's redemptive love, but when along the developmental pathway do we believe God's concern for a person's eschatological destiny begins? Is it at conception? Is it at four days, ten days, or fourteen days?

Though we do not appeal to it as a foundation for a theologically informed assessment of the cloning and stem cell debates, we find the fourteen-day rule to be more persuasive than arguments for conception. It is sufficiently convincing to warrant support as a subpremise within the larger beneficence framework. One can fully understand and appreciate Pope John Paul II and others who are convinced that dignity begins at conception; yet a closer look at what science tells us about embryo development makes the gastrulation threshold more defensible. (One can, by the way, hold to the fourteen-day rule and still hold to a prolife position on abortion.)

The belief that the embryo should be protected from the moment of conception is argued in various ways. Two arguments appear frequently. First is the argument from potential. This is the argument appealed to by the Kass council majority. The majority points to the seamless trajectory of development from conception to birth. In light of this continuum, the Kass council holds the conceptus to be nascent human life and deserving of a "shared obligation to protect it."[28]

As many supporters of embryonic stem cell research have rightly pointed out, the argument from potentiality assesses the status of the embryo in accordance with the presumption that the embryo can and will be placed in vivo. Stem cell research is conducted on embryos in vitro. The potential for an embryo in the lab to become a baby is nil. This is not a criticism, moral concession, or an argument from geography (as critics rhetorically put it). It is an ethically relevant fact. An embryo in vitro has many intrinsic qualities that are needed for baby making, but it does not have all of the necessary qualities. Although it has DNA, at minimum it still needs a womb to proceed down the developmental pathway.

The second argument is that articulated by the Vatican in *Donum Vitae*. This argument holds that with conception a genuinely new human individual comes into existence. When this argument appeals to genetic novelty for support, it fails to account for current embryology. It makes little sense to associate the appearance of the individual with novel DNA. If the existence of twins had not already made this clear, the birth of Dolly should certainly put the matter to rest.

It is difficult to hold to the fourteen-day rule with the same level of dogmatic fervor that the pope, and by implication, that the Kass council holds to conception; it is subject to changes in perspective as embryology expands our knowledge. It is a finite human judgment call to combine beneficence with the fourteen-day rule when orienting public policy.

The recognition of the finitude of our ethical judgments could be incorporated into both sides in the stem cell or therapeutic cloning controversy. Science alone does not tell us when morally protectable personhood begins. We bring our ethical criteria for personhood to the science, to be molded,

confirmed, or disconfirmed. Science itself plays the limited role of corrobo-
rator or critic.

In granting that the science of embryology in itself cannot supply the decisive biological fact that resolves the debate between the Vatican protection
of the fertilized egg and the fourteen-day rule, the policy decision we would
make here would have to take the form of an ethical leap of faith. In making this leap, we could imagine some sort of "better-safe-than-sorry" principle being invoked. The embryo protection position as defended by the Vatican and by the Kass council's majority might say, When in doubt about the
moral status of the blastocyst, it is safer to assume it has protectable duty and
avoid doing harm. In contrast, the Singapore BAC report and the minority
within the U.S. report might say, When in doubt about the moral status of the
blastocyst, it is safer to assume the appropriateness of the fourteen-day rule and
proceed with this potentially life-saving and life-enhancing research. The former would appeal primarily to nonmaleficence, the latter to beneficence.

If the Vatican could convince us beyond a doubt to support its position
regarding morally protectable dignity at conception, this would be sufficient
to persuade us to join the antitherapeutic-cloning forces. The fourteen-day
rule, to our reading, however, holds at least equal if not superior merit, even
if it falls short of being absolutely decisive. Our fundamental commitment is
to beneficence. So, in order to be safe rather than sorry (vis-à-vis the potential risk of failing to act decisively on behalf those suffering from degenera-
tive diseases), we join with those who wish to encourage stem cell and related research on the grounds that there exists here a potential for future
healing that will relieve human suffering on a large scale. To elect an unsure
commitment to nonmaleficence rather than an unsure commitment to
beneficence would be, as in Jesus' parable of the Good Samaritan, passing by
on the other side.

This amounts to a contingent ethical argument in support of laboratory
research on therapies employing stem cells and cloning. While affirming this
contingent ethical judgment, we remain somewhat unsatisfied about unfinished theological business. Despite all we said in our introduction regarding
the important role that eschatology should play in defining human life, we
find ourselves arguing along with everyone else in the archonic playground.
For the sake of the public policy debate, we find ourselves conceding that biological origin—whether at conception or at adherence to the mother's
uterus—determines moral status. Within the framework of the archonic assumptions, we believe the fourteen-day rule edges out the moment of con-

ception position, and we still more earnestly believe that beneficence should be given larger place in ethical argumentation.

Notes

1. Bioethics Advisory Committee Singapore (hereinafter BAC), *Ethical, Legal and Social Issues in Human Stem Cell Research, Reproductive and Therapeutic Cloning.* Report submitted to the Ministerial Committee for Life Sciences, June 2002. And President's Council on Bioethics, *Human Cloning and Human Dignity: An Ethical Inquiry.* Report submitted to U.S. President George W. Bush, 10 July 2002.

2. Ian Wilmut, along with Donald Bruce, describe current nuclear transfer technology as a hit-and-miss affair; and the Roslin Institute has declared that cloning human beings is ethically unacceptable. See Wilmut and Bruce, "Dolly Mixture," in Donald Bruce and Ann Bruce, eds., *Engineering Genesis: The Ethics of Genetic Engineering in Non-Human Species* (London: Earthscan Publications, 1998), 71–76.

3. "The principle of beneficence in its simplest form is that we ought to do good or, if expressed as an obligation, that there is an obligation to help others." Marvin Kohl, "Beneficence," in Lawrence C. Becker and Charlotte B. Becker, *Encyclopedia of Ethics,* 2d ed., 3 vols. (New York: Routledge, 2001), 1:128.

4. Congregation for the Doctrine of the Faith, *Donum Vitae* (Vatican City, 1987), in Thomas A. Shannon, ed., *Bioethics* (New York: Paulist Press, 1987); also available at www.vatican.va.

5. Immanuel Kant, *Groundwork for the Metaphysics of Morals*, ed. and trans. H. J. Patton (New York: Harper, 1948).

6. Knud Løgstrup, "The Radical Character of the Demand and the Social Norms," in Hans Fink and Alasdair MacIntyre, eds., *The Ethical Demand* (Notre Dame, Ind.: University of Notre Dame Press, 1997), 44–63.

7. BAC, iv.

8. BAC, vii.

9. Ibid.

10. Ibid.

11. See, *Human Cloning and Human Dignity: The Report of the President's Council on Bioethics,* Foreword by Leon R. Kass (New York: PublicAffairs, 2002).

12. Leon R. Kass and James Q. Wilson, *The Ethics of Human Cloning* (Washington D.C.: AEI Press, 1998).

13. Kass report, iii.

14. Ibid., xvii.

15. Ibid., xvii–xviii.

16. Ibid., xviii.

17. Ibid., xix.

18. Ibid.

19. Ibid.

20. Ibid.
21. Ibid.
22. Ibid., xx.
23. Ibid.
24. Ibid.
25. Ibid.
26. Ibid.
27. Ibid.
28. Ibid., xx.

NINE

Human Embryonic Stem Cell Research: Ethics in the Face of Uncertainty

KEVIN T. FITZGERALD, S.J.

Too often the opposing positions in the stem cell and cloning debate are presented in terms of the obviousness of the assertions they make. In light of the complex nature of these controversial issues challenging our society, the reality that informs these assertions is much less clear and certain than the debaters themselves often recognize. Therefore, this essay addresses the question of how we might best respond to the challenge of human embryonic stem cell research in the face of the uncertainties that pervade this issue.

Uncertainty is present in all aspects of this issue: scientific, medical, moral, religious, and political. This essay begins with the areas of uncertainty that are perhaps most surprising and, hence, most vexing for those engaged in this public debate—the scientific and the medical.

The Scientific Setting

In order to appreciate fully the scientific and medical uncertainties in stem cell research, it is helpful to put the science of stem cell research within a larger context of the current advances in molecular and cellular biology. Stem cells are only one part of the rapidly expanding arena of molecular biology research. This arena includes such topics as genetic therapies, genomics, pharmacology, proteomics, and various types of cellular and tissue research.[1] All of these research trajectories offer tremendous potential for advancing our scientific knowledge as well as the possibility of leading to new and exciting medical therapies and products.

A couple of examples may help give a sense of the scope of these possibilities. Much has been written in both academic journals and the popular press about the promise of human gene therapy. Until recently there has been little concrete evidence of the fulfillment of that promise, and, instead, we have witnessed some tragic and troubling results.[2] The latest results of some clinical trials employing gene therapies to treat immune system disorders, however, indicate that the promise might be at least partially realized.[3]

In these clinical experiments, the researchers added a functioning gene to the cells of individuals who were diseased because of a defect in one of their genes. The drawbacks to this approach include the problems of not being able to control where the new gene incorporates itself in a cell's DNA and that of the mutated gene remaining in the cells. In the near future, researchers hope to address these problems by directly replacing or repairing the diseased genes.[4]

If the disease to be treated results from flaws in a region of DNA much larger than a single nucleotide or even a single gene, researchers may try to employ artificial chromosomes to address the situation. Artificial chromosomes are able to carry several new genes, perhaps many of them, into the cells of the patients' bodies. In addition to this larger genetic carrying capacity, human artificial chromosomes may have the advantages of maintaining a more stable number of the copies of a gene within a cell and better control of long-term gene expression.[5] Using these genetic technologies to target both small and large genetic mutations, in the future physicians may have much greater success in treating the genetic causes of many diseases.

If these genetic technologies can be used successfully to treat disease, however, might they not also be used to change the genetic constitution of a human being in order to alter an individual's physical or behavioral characteristics? Would changing an individual's genetic constitution to include DNA sequences that are not known to have been present in any human being before change the human nature of that individual? Is there an amount or kind of alteration that would result in an individual no longer being human?

These examples from human genetic engineering have been used to show that the ethical challenges generated by cutting-edge biotechnologies are very much the same as those raised by human stem cell research. An example from stem cell research will help demonstrate this point. In an experiment designed to investigate the emergence of reservoirs of neural stem cells in the developing fetal brain, Evan Snyder and Curt Freed directed research whereby cells from a neural stem cell line derived from a human fetal cadaver were implanted into the developing brain of a fetal bonnet monkey at approximately twelve to thirteen weeks of gestation. After sacrificing the fetal monkey four weeks later, Freed and Snyder found that the human neural stem cells had migrated and incorporated into the fetal monkey brain.[6]

Although it was not the stated purpose of the experiment, these results pose serious questions about the uniqueness or significance of human nature. If human beings are considerably interchangeable with other animals on a cellular and/or genetic level, how might that reality affect our concepts of ourselves? If we have the ability to interchange genes or cells or even tissues and organs with other animals, at what point does an addition of nonhuman cells, for example, make a human being someone or something else?

The experiment with human neural stem cells in fetal monkey brains is particularly relevant to these questions, because arguments are often presented that focus on the human brain as the physiological basis for what makes human beings special or unique. If cells from humans and other animals can be mixed early in development and still form a functioning brain, then does it—will it—should it matter what percentage of a brain is made up of human cells? Perhaps, instead, research will indicate that the timing of a genetic or cellular manipulation during organismal development is more important than the amount of material inserted? Whatever the case may be, brain experiments mixing cells from different species will certainly add to the challenges scientific research is raising to our commonly held concepts of what it means to be human and what makes humans special, if anything. In light of these challenges and the troubling ramifications they may have for our moral frameworks and ethical reasoning, because of their unsettling effects on our beliefs and concepts about human nature and human value, one could easily ask why such research is being done at all.

One can easily project several important goals for research using these amazing cells. Often these goals are grouped into three categories: basic research in human development, safer and more specific drug development, and therapies to repair or replace damaged tissues and organs.[7] The basic research is obviously significant because scientists want to understand better how human beings develop from a single cellular structure to the complex structure of an adult body. In addition, because stem cells function to replace the cells we lose in daily life, basic stem cell research may help answer questions about disease, injury, and aging.

The goal of safer and more specific drug development is one that might be less obvious to the public at large. The idea here is to use stem cells from different individuals to grow cells, tissues, or perhaps even organs. Then instead of, or in addition to, testing drugs on animals or generic human cell lines that may not represent accurately or precisely the reactions of a target human tissue, the cells or tissues grown from different individuals can be tested for the efficacy and toxicity of various drugs. From such research, companies might get a much better idea of which individuals would benefit more from which drugs, and which individuals should avoid which drugs, even before clinical trials with human subjects are begun.

Eventually, the goal of this research is to develop products and therapies that would allow physicians to become more direct, efficient, and effective in replacing and repairing the cells, tissues, and organs of an individual that may have been damaged or destroyed. This medical approach is now being promoted as "regenerative medicine."[8] In the public debate surrounding the stem cell issue, it is most often this goal of using stem cell research to regenerate tissues and organs that receives the greatest attention.

Benefits, Harms, and Uncertainty

The public debate concerning human embryonic stem cells revolves around weighing the good of doing this scientific research, with the primary goal of medical benefit, against the harms involved in doing research on human embryos. Having listed some of the benefits of this research above, I now turn briefly to the harms involved.

The most obvious harm cited in the public debate, and probably the most broadly contentious, is the destruction of the human embryo. This issue becomes exacerbated when proposals are made for intentionally creating human embryos, either by in vitro fertilization or by nuclear transfer techniques (cloning), in order to destroy them for their embryonic stem cells. At issue here is the value—moral, legal, and social—societies are to acknowledge in or give to human embryos. The different arguments made concerning the value of human embryos range from claiming that they should be treated basically the same as any piece of human tissue to claiming that they should be treated basically the same as any human person. Because much has already been written across this broad spectrum, I wish to address only one aspect of the debate that highlights the uncertainty involved in this issue—the ambiguities encountered in this debate concerning the term "embryo."

In order to support the claim that human embryos should not have protections similar to those held by human subjects in general, it is often argued that the relatively high rate of embryo loss in early pregnancy (with some estimates at 50 percent[9]) indicates that embryos should receive a lesser moral and legal status than human subjects in general.[10] Otherwise, it is asked, why do not societies and cultures encourage the ritual mourning of the loss of these embryos, and why do they not advocate greater medical interventions to save these human lives? Prescinding from an analysis of differing traditions concerning the appropriate response to death early in human development, one can, instead, evaluate the importance of this argument by focusing on the ambiguity, or even equivocation, inherent in this argument with respect to the use of the term "embryo."

When one argues about the ethical status of a human embryo, the underlying reality about which one is arguing can be described as that stage of human development we all transited on our way to our current stage of human development, whatever that may be. In other words, we are discussing human embryos in the context of what we ourselves once were. This context is not the same as the scientific one that undergirds the statistics about human embryo losses in early pregnancy. Such statistics might readily include abnormal growths, such as complete hydatidiform moles.[11] Though hydatidiform moles may have characteristics similar to embryos, these growths are not developing along the trajectory of a human organism. Rather, these growths are disorganized in their development to the extent that they may require surgical removal in order to prevent them from becoming life-threatening cancers. The question then arises: in light of the possibility of nonembryonic pregnancies, how many of these pregnancy losses are actually human embryos of the type we envision in our ethical debates and how many are nonembryonic pregnancies? Once again, it appears that we are confronted with significant uncertainty. Because our scientific conceptualizations of an embryo may not match the embryo conceptualizations employed in our ethical analyses, the relevance of the argument regarding the percentages of embryos lost in pregnancy may be only minimal at best with respect to the human embryo research debate.

This problem of uncertainty in arguing about the ethical status of embryos fits within the larger context of uncertainty about human nature described earlier in this essay. It is not surprising that there is difficulty in defining the beginnings of human life, if it is indeed becoming more difficult to define human life itself because of our rapidly increasing scientific information. From this larger context, these uncertainties in the definition and understanding of embryos and human life may help to explain the impasse currently experienced in the human embryo research debates. If different, and even contrary, understandings of the beginnings of human life are being used in this public debate, then without extensive clarifications a resolution of this contentious issue may be improbable if not impossible. And if we cannot reach resolution on the status of the human embryo, how will we as a society address the coming dilemmas surrounding our concepts of human life or human nature?

I have argued elsewhere that the answers to these profound questions will require a revitalization of the philosophical anthropologies that undergird our ethical systems as well as our concepts of health, disease, and human nature.[12] This revitalization will likely entail broad interdisciplinary and intercultural dialogue and, hence, some length of time. Still, as our society currently wrestles with these more fundamental questions, one needs to ask what our society is doing now to resolve the debate concerning human embryonic research in spite of its contentiousness and the uncertainty surrounding it.

In one sense, this dilemma is not new for us, because as a society we have already decided that, in light of past abuses such as the research performed on African Americans or the mentally disabled, it is sometimes best to limit what science and technology can do in order to better serve what is good for society.[13] In view of the harms caused to people in the name of scientific or medical progress, our society and others around the world have created guidelines and agencies to protect human research subjects from undue risks and harms.[14] This protection of human research subjects is an ongoing process, with new revelations and investigations regularly being reported by government commissions and the media.[15] The controversies surrounding human embryo research not only involve the debate over the status of human embryos, but also include other human subject issues such as the procurement of human eggs in large numbers as might be required by nuclear transfer research and technology.[16]

From within this current context of protections from undue research risk and harm, how is our current system of public ethical reflection responding to the human embryo research predicament? One response to this contentious social issue has been for various organizations to gather panels of experts to investigate, analyze, and evaluate the issue with the goal of generating recommendations for actions to be undertaken by governmental and/or other agencies. In general, the arguments and recommendations formulated by these expert panels have been reflective of or employed by many who are engaged in the broader public debate, especially with regard to legislation that has been or is to be addressed on both the state and national levels. The arguments that have been made in support of human embryo research often fall into two primary categories, referred to here as "need" and "number."[17] A brief analysis of these arguments will reveal the uncertainties inherent in them and, consequently, their insufficiency to serve as justifications for pursuing this socially contentious research.

Addressing the argument of the *need* for human embryo research, it is important to recall that, as was observed in the beginning of this essay, the diseases suggested as likely targets for human embryonic stem cell research are also being targeted by researchers using other approaches, such as genetic therapies, drug development, and adult stem cells. It may well be the case that for many patients the treatments for their illnesses may come more quickly from research avenues other than human embryonic stem cell research and that these alternative treatments may even be better than any treatment derived from human embryonic stem cell research.

In response to this uncertainty as to what line of research might yet prove most successful in meeting the medical needs of people afflicted with severe or fatal diseases, proponents of human embryo research have argued that all scientifically sound lines of research should be pursued simultaneously, so we have the best chance of discovering what will work as soon as possible. From a scientific perspective, this approach makes the most sense. In science, when there is uncertainty, one does all the research indicated to gain the desired knowledge and understanding. As was observed above, however, what is best for science is not always best for a society and its members. Some lines of research may be restricted or banned, regardless of their scientific appeal, in order to protect the well-being of a society. Research that is as controversial and contentious as human embryo research must have reasons to justify its pursuit that are as ethically compelling as the harms it creates.

At this point in the debate, human embryo research proponents often turn to the second argument cited above and emphasize the incredible *number* of people who could potentially benefit from such research. These proponents can point to the uncertainty inherent in all this biological research and argue that no society should deny people who suffer from severe and fatal diseases the potential benefits of this research, even if the research is controversial and contentious within a given society. Associating this research with the substantial societal value of medical healing gives this argument significance.

There is, however, a fundamental flaw in this argument that undermines its power and claim. The flaw lies in its assumption of a direct correlation between scientific or medical advance and medical benefit for those who need it. The realities of health care systems both in our own society and around the world argue against this assumption. With respect to health care in the United States, we need to acknowledge that, even if treatments from human embryonic stem cell research are the first to be proven successful, many if not most people who need these treatments will not get them.

Evidence of the accuracy of this bleak assessment of our health care system is found in the December 2001 report of the President's Cancer Panel. Although great strides have been made in cancer research during the past three decades of our war on cancer, the panel concludes, "In short, our health care system is broken, and it is failing people with cancer and those at risk for cancer—all of us."[18] Worldwide the situation is much more bleak, considering that millions of children die each year from a lack of clean water, not to mention inadequate access to minimal health care technology.[19] Therefore, just because many people in the world might tragically share a devastating disease, such as diabetes or Parkinson's, one cannot conclude that this tragedy will be resolved by breakthroughs in research. The greater tragedy is that only a relative few will reap the benefits of many of our medical research advances. The argument from *number* does not fit our social reality.

At this juncture, it is critical that the arguments from uncertainty presented above be applied precisely. These arguments have been made to call attention to the flaws in the reasoning often presented in support of human embryonic research. These arguments do not argue against the pursuit of medical advances *per se*. These arguments do, however, place scientific and medical research in the larger context of the good of societies in general. The National Bioethics Advisory Commission acknowledged the importance of this context and the consequent requirement for greater justification than normal in pursuing scientific research that is socially contentious.[20] Therefore, if the justification for proceeding with the destruction of human embryos for research rests even in part on these claims of *need* and *number*, this justification is flawed and requires rethinking.

The evidence and analysis put forward in this essay attest to the pervasiveness of *uncertainty* in all of the aspects of the human embryo research issue. This uncertainty, it has been argued, even undermines the proposals for pursuing this research put forth by some of the expert panels commissioned to address this issue.

How then should society proceed? The arguments of this essay suggest two responses that could be implemented immediately within the current circumstances of our society. First, in recognition of the need for research into stem cell biology in order to understand better its promises and perils for future societal decisions, governmental support should be increased for stem cell research using animal models and nonembryonic human stem cells. This response would achieve scientific progress without raising especially contentious social and ethical concerns.

Second, in recognition of the vast numbers of people, within our own nation and around the world, who suffer from severe and lethal diseases or injuries, the findings and recommendations for improving health care proposed by expert groups such as the President's Cancer Panel and the World Health Organization should receive at least the same level of attention and action as has been expended on human embryo research.

Notes

1. The National Center for Biotechnology Information has web sites that provide an overview of many of these technologies and Internet links to other resources explaining these technologies. See both www.ncbi.nlm.nih.gov/About/primer/index.html and www.ncbi.nlm.nih.gov/About/outreach/index.html [accessed 5 January 2003].

2. See N. Somia and I. M. Verma, "Gene Therapy: Trials and Tribulations," *Nature Review Genetics,* vol. 1, no. 2 (November 2000): 91–99; and D. Teichler Zallen, "US Gene Therapy in Crisis," *Trends in Genetics,* vol. 16, no. 6 (June 2000): 272–75.

3. F. S. Rosen, "Successful Gene Therapy for Severe Combined Immunodeficiency," *New England Journal of Medicine,* vol. 346, no. 16 (18 April 2002): 1241–43; and S. Hacein-Bey-Abina, F. Le Deist, F. Carlier, C. Bouneaud, C. Hue, J. P. De Villartay, A. J. Thrasher, N. Wulffraat, R. Sorensen, S. Dupuis-Girod, A. Fischer, E. G. Davies, W. Kuis, L. Leiva, and M. Cavazzana-Calvo, "Sustained Correction of X-Linked Severe Combined Immunodeficiency by Ex Vivo Gene Therapy," *New England Journal of Medicine,* vol. 346, no. 16 (18 April 2002): 1185–93.

4. Gene replacement could involve techniques known as homologous recombination, while gene repair could be done using techniques that correct a mutation by replacing the single letter (nucleotide) that is misspelled in the DNA. For example, see P. D. Richardson, L. B. Augustin, B. T. Kren, and C. J. Steer, "Gene Repair and Transposon-Mediated Gene Therapy," *Stem Cells,* vol. 20, no. 2 (March 2002): 105–18.

5. H. F. Willard, "Artificial Chromosomes Coming to Life," *Science,* vol. 290 (2000): 1308–9.

6. V. Ourednik, J. Ourednik, J. D. Flax, W. M. Zawada, C. Hutt, C. Yang, K. I. Park, S. U. Kim, R. L. Sidman, C. R. Freed, and E. Y. Snyder, "Segregation of Human Neural Stem Cells in the Developing Primate Forebrain," *Science,* vol. 293, no. 5536 (September 2001): 1820–24.

7. See the National Institutes of Health stem cell primer webpage, www4.od.nih.gov/stemcell/figure5.jpg [accessed 5 January 2003].

8. For background on stem cell biology and the perspective of the National Research Council committee on stem cell research, see their report, *Stem Cells and the Future of*

Regenerative Medicine, which can be found online at www.nap.edu/books/0309076307 /html/ [accessed 5 January 2003].

9. For more on miscarriage and its causes, see the March of Dimes website, www. modimes.org/HealthLibrary/334_592.htm [accessed 5 January 2003].

10. For two examples of this type of argument, see Jeffrey Spike, "Bush and Stem Cell Research: An Ethically Confused Policy," and Robert Baker, "Stem Cell Rhetoric and the Pragmatics of Naming," both in *American Journal of Bioethics,* vol. 2, no. 1 (2002): 45 and 53, respectively.

11. For more on molar pregnancies, see www.modimes.org/HealthLibrary/ [accessed 5 January 2003].

12. Kevin T. FitzGerald, "Philosophical Anthropologies and the HGP," in Phillip R. Sloan, ed., *Controlling Our Destinies: The Human Genome Project from Historical, Philosophical, Social, and Ethical Perspectives* (Notre Dame, Ind.: Notre Dame University Press, 2000), 395–410.

13. Adil E. Shamoo and Joan L. O'Sullivan, "The Ethics of Research on the Mentally Disabled," in John F. Monagle and David C. Thomasma, eds., *Health Care Ethics: Critical Issues for the Twenty-first Century* (Gaithersburg, Md.: Aspen Publishers, 1998): 239–50.

14. Guidelines for protecting human research subjects are found in such reports as the World Medical Association's "Declaration of Helsinki," and the U.S. "Protection of Human Subjects," *Code of Federal Regulations* 45 CFR 46, revised March 8, 1983, as well as the Recombinant DNA Advisory Committee, Office of Human Research Protections, and so forth.

15. Examples of current events include the Virginia governor's apology for forced sterilizations (www.governor.state.va.us/Press_Policy/Releases/May2002/May0202.htm [accessed 5 January 2003]) and recent U.S. Navy bioweapon exposures reports (www. cbsnews.com/stories/2002/05/24/national/main510079.shtml [accessed 5 January 2003).

16. Andrew Pollack, "Use of Cloning to Tailor Treatment Has Big Hurdles, Including Cost," *New York Times* (December 18, 2001), F2, 1.

17. Although many examples of these basic arguments can be found in the transcripts of congressional and state legislative hearings, one can find the arguments from need and number clearly stated in the following documents from three of the highest profile expert panels assembled to date: American Association for the Advancement of Science and the Institute for Civil Society report, "Stem Cell Research and Applications: Monitoring the Frontiers of Biomedical Research" (www.aaas.org/spp/sfrl/projects/stem/main.html [accessed 5 January 2003]); National Bioethics Advisory Commission report, "Ethical Issues in Human Stem Cell Research, September 1999" (http://bioethics.georgetown. edu/nbac/pubs.html [accessed 5 January 2003]); and the National Research Council and Institute of Medicine report: "Stem Cells and the Future of Regenerative Medicine (2002)" (http://books.nap.edu/books/0309076307/html /R1.html [accessed 5 January 2003]).

18. President's Cancer Panel report (December 2001), "Voices of a Broken System: Real People, Real Problems," 2 (http://deainfo.nci.nih.gov/ADVISORY/pcp/video-summary.htm [accessed 5 January 2003]).

19. World Health Organization, "Children's Environmental Health" (www.who. int/peh/ceh/index.htm [accessed 5 January 2003]).

20. National Bioethics Advisory Commission report, n. 18, pp. 52–53.

TEN

Freedoms, Duties, and Limits: The Ethics of Research in Human Stem Cells

LAURIE ZOLOTH

To think about ethics and moral philosophy in medicine is to imagine ourselves at a crossroads, a turning point, a pivotal moment in history and science. It is intensely interesting and therefore frequently insisted on that we are heroic actors, all of us, facing a choice that will change the world as we know it. It is comforting to know that this image is not novel. In fact, the sense of standing at a turning point and being faced with competing moral appeals and competing truth claims is the archetypal scene of moral philosophy itself. We are indeed at a crossroads in medicine as we face the decisions of stem cell research. Here, when we meet to discuss the tantalizing promise of research, we do so on ground that is crossed by many possible roads, each with a long beginning.

But is it new to be standing on the open ground of despair in the face of illness and frailty, to be yearning for understanding as we stand by the bedside of a dying child? Hardly—it is the oldest of griefs. Is it new to be worried as we intervene in the world, and as our science obliterates a fundamental fixity of what we think to be natural, turning night into day with electricity, turning pain into oblivion with anesthesia, turning illness into resistance with vaccines? Hardly. Our worry about the use and misuse of forbidden knowledge is the oldest of terrors.

That the terrain on which we debate stem cell research is familiar, however, does not make it easier to navigate. In fact, stem cell research, a technology barely out of the box, is one of the most fervently debated ethical issues of our day, the subject taken up by the United Nations, fourteen international and two American bioethics commissions, the U.S. Senate and House, and two administrations, not to mention nearly every major religious organization and patient care advocacy group. This occurs, I would argue, because embryonic stem cell research reawakens some core debates about ourselves, debates about who we are and what we are intended to do, core debates about the nature of the self and the duty to the other, the creature that is humanity and our frail creaturely being, and the vastness of our power and hence our responsibilities.

Starting on Common Ground

Because this is an article about what questions divide us, let us start in a more promising place: what could we agree on? Are there ethical norms that would be helpful in thinking about the ethics of controversial science? In a pluralistic society, in the presence of new science, and in the face of moral discord, bioethics aims to carefully consider different moral appeals.

First, we could say that, in our American democracy, basic research science is an open question and, like any open intellectual question, it needs protection to be freely asked and pursued. We could agree that basic research is a kind of free speech, and we would want it to be spoken unencumbered, like all ideas in the academy, free from the manipulation or particular use of state authority or the power of any one established religion. We understand and like our scientists to be alert to the world in its entirety and variety, to be free to think—anything. Free inquiry is the basis for the scientific method itself.

Second, we could agree that health care research is a public good and hence needs to be freely witnessed, discussed, and debated in our democracy without secrecy and deception. If research is free speech and hence entitled to its protections, we have a duty to speak in a way that can be answered. We like our scientist to tell us, and right away, the witnessing, watching citizens, what they are up to and to explain how it might be applied so we can understand what the stakes are for us as citizens.

Third, medicine and, hence, health care research are vivid moral gestures made in response to a world of suffering. Basic science is driven by many motives, including the purely Baconian pursuit to see how the world is put together, but medical research aims at more than this curiosity. It is morally warranted, indeed called into being precisely by our mutual vulnerability and as a mutual response to the need of the suffering other. It is ethical because it is about the way we hear and then struggle to answer the call of our neighbor. We want our research, when it is applied, to result in a world that is more compassionate, more just, and more fully expressive of human beauty. We want health care to be beneficent.

Fourth, we want research to be careful. We do worry that the moral gesture itself, and more deeply we worry that applications of science, might hurt a world already shaken by powerful human intervention. We want to be able to say "no," or "slow down," to some research, limiting the power to put all knowledge into practice. We want, in short, research that is free, good, fair, and careful—analogs to the classic principle of bioethics—autonomous, beneficent, nonmaleficent, and just.

Finally, we cannot fully agree on the question of when human personhood begins or ends, for this is essentially a question of faith. My interpretive community of Jewish scholars understands the blastocyst that is developed by artificial means in a petri dish—one that will never be near a woman's womb, and in the first week of its development— to be a possibility, unformed and not ensouled. But a possible thing is not the same as the thing itself, and we treat each being relative to our duties at that time. We can agree, for example, that with utter certainty each of us will become a corpse, yet we do not treat one another as corpses. We can develop some sense of overlapping consensus, and we can agree, for the most part, on boundary conditions within this consensus. The fundamental moral differences between how the Sharia law of Islam, the talmudic textual reasoning of a Jew, and the principles by which many Protestants understand moral status of embryos and the position of many Roman Catholics and other Protestants at this time will not be a point of agreement. This was not the case prior to the middle of the 1800s, and it may not be the case at some later point in history, but we stand at this place in time, and for now we stand in fundamentally different positions on this matter. While I hear the gravity of the Roman Catholic concern for the developing life and honor that gravity, it will not convince me toward a different understanding of my Jewish position on what a blastocyst is and what our duties toward it are.

In fact, it has been the issue of moral status put forward by the churches that has dominated our American discourse. The problem of deep disagreements of faith will continue to vex the issue of the moral status of the human blastocyst. This is a critical problem for a polity facing collective decisions, to be sure, but it is surely not the only issue that faces us when we ponder research in this field. Although the question of the embryo is critical, this question of origins cannot be allowed to obscure other arguments or divert us from other questions. Some other arguments are equally urgent and equally emergent from the most sincere location of faith. They, too, need to be more fully elaborated. These arguments emerge from Jewish ethics, which has a stance of cautious optimism about human stem cell research. I argue here that what is at stake for us is not the moral status of the five-day-old blastocyst, about which we cannot agree, but the moral status of ourselves as we perform, witness, and learn about human stem cell research. All of us, as we stand in the public square, participate in the activity, the doing or the undoing of it, and we are witnesses to the history and the future we create at this moment. There is no null position.

Premises and Duties

In thinking about the ethical issues in stem cell research, we are drawn to organize the conundrums into questions of origin and status, questions of process and fair use of subjects, and questions of telos, or goals and ends of the work. Let me argue that we first need to confront a primary task—the one of establishing the first premises of how we regard these questions—of who we need to become as a people to address our future coherently, courageously, and morally.

Bioethics often asks the question, What is the right act, and what makes it so? In this, we often ask about consequences: If we do this act, what will happen? Will we be more or less happy? Utilitarian considerations drive the debate. My arguments ask another question: What are our essential deontological constraints prior to doing the action? What are our duties, and how does the performance of these duties create in us our character? It is the question of Aristotle and of Alexis deTocqeville, asking us about the habits of the heart. So who are we? How are we shaped by our decisions? To what do we aspire? Let me suggest six such duties.

Justice

First, we are makers of justice. This moral consideration is often left to the end of the discussion, and yet it is a central concern in bioethics, so let me begin with it. Stem cell research raises considerable questions of justice, both in basic research and in the applications of the research. What is the moral status of the community? Does the research pursuit help us to create a world that is more just? I would argue that it does. The arguments are best articulated in European ethics debates. Unlike American principles of ethics, the ethics of Europeans name "attention to the vulnerable" and "a commitment to solidarity" as core values.

A just community is best judged as such by such commitments: stem cell research must be structured so that it is directed to helping the vulnerable and to improving the essential social contract. And nowhere is the social contract more frayed and at risk than in the health care system, a system in which nearly forty-five million American citizens have no assured access to health care services. All research (stem cells being merely the last in line to be so queried) must aim at increasing access to basic, decent, universally available health care. Allocation of health care funding must be fair in both procedure and substance, and innovations in research must be made for the maximum benefit of a larger polity.

Stem cells are intriguing to justice theorists for precisely the same reason that they are intriguing to the market. They represent a therapeutic intervention that, unlike heart transplants, could be universally available, replicable, and scaleable. If the daunting problems of histocompatibility can be overcome, embryonic stem cells could be made universally accessible to anybody. Unlike adult stem cells, which would have to be created each time for each particular user, the premise of application for embryonic stem cells is the wide use. Bioethicists defend high-intensity interventions like organ transplant, which have saved, albeit at high cost, thousands of individuals. But organ transplants are terribly expensive and always rationed, and the risk entailed means that the vast numbers of people with chronic disease ought not undergo such a risk. Stem cell therapy is aimed at a wider community of vulnerable patients, and at no one particular category, age, ethnicity, or class. The sort of injury and diseases that stem cells are indicated for are not boutique, or rare. On the contrary, cell death and cell growth are at the core of nearly all disorders. Research into these essential causes would be precisely the sort of research we ought to insist on.

Further, understanding how embryonic cells are programmed and reprogrammed might allow us to understand how to deprogram cells, allowing adult cells to regenerate, teaching the body to heal itself. The demand for justice and the scrutiny that genetic medicine is given are indications that we understand the power of genetics to reconfigure the self and the society. In this way, the very debate about stem cells forces precisely the justice considerations that I would argue must be a part of medicine. The principle of justice places a priority on the public aspects of research, on public funding and on public oversight review boards for protocols.

Moral Discernment

We have a duty to be discerning. Human persons are moral actors. We are made as namers of the world, created with a curiosity to know and judge and decide. Moral discernment is the way we become human. For religious philosophers from the Abramic tradition, it is the making of covenants, social contracts, and the taking of law that marks the beginning of social authority. These social abilities create the scaffold of communities governed by law and not by hierarchies, somewhat the way that the framers of the U.S. Constitution understood this duty. As law receivers and the judges of human events, we live in history and are responsible to it. Using judgment and debate, we move to make decisions on the natural order of the world. We create and live by laws. We give voting privileges to some and not others. We decide when teenagers are competent to exercise specific rights; and we can make judgments, finally, on when human life begins. We modify and change our law when the facts of the case change, when new things are understood, and new abilities emerge. Our duty to judge answers the critique that we cannot stop evil consequences of research, that we will unthinkingly tumble down every available slippery slope, that we are unable to erect fences, norms, and rules to protect women, or gametes, or children. We have a duty to judge, and to say "no," or what are ethicists for? We can say "no" to reproductive cloning but not to research cloning, just as we say "no" to selling organs but not to donating organs, or "no" to slavery but not to graduate school.

Healing and Caring

We have a duty to heal the ill and save lives if we can and to care for them if we cannot. It is this duty that animates Jewish advocacy of medical research. It is an overriding a priori duty, taking precedence over other ritual or practical obligations, like the Sabbath observance. This obligation is not only a Jewish premise, it is one of the internal and intrinsic goals of medicine and, as I noted above, one of the goals of medical research. But here I want to extend this duty, and I would argue that it also ought to be an ethical goal of a minimally decent civil society as well. It is regrettable that this duty tends to be isolated and given to others, to physicians and the dwindling supply of nurses. The taking on of this obligation to one's neighbor broadens our understanding of both who the neighbor is supposed to be to us and who we are supposed to be to the neighbor. In the philosophy of Emmanuel Levinas, I am transformed by my duty to answer the call of the neighbor, "I am the one who must come up with the goods."

For Levinas, we must answer the call to help and heal with our entire social goods, with our bodies if need be, with the skin of ourselves. My life is defined by my service to the vulnerable. What might occur in the debate if we took this philosophic claim to heart? It might help us to understand that altruism is a good and a possible human endeavor and see the moral virtue of gifts instead of fearing coercion or worrying about ownership and property at every step of the process. The moral universe is so constituted as to be unstable, violent, and failed that we must take this step toward the other if we are to make ourselves whole. In fact, it is this radical recognition of utter responsibility that allows us to break out of the paralyzing and deadening idea that the pain of the other is not my problem, that it can be simply ignored without peril to myself. What would I sacrifice to heal the other in need? What do I place before that need? The researcher and the patients and the doctors and the nurses must ask, What is my moral status? How am I acting toward my neighbor?

Tending and Transforming

We are guardians, watchmen of a world that is incomplete. It is a Jewish argument that creation is not complete. If it were, in the arguments of the Talmud, loaves of bread and suits of linen would dangle from stalks of wheat and flax. But they do not—we live in a world we are commanded to tend and transform, and the bread we eat we are commanded to pull from the natural earth in a transforming act. Human persons are defined by a duty to finish and repair a broken and incomplete nature world, a world that is interrupted, filled with many unfinished tasks. Nature is not sacred and not inviolate. It needs human actions to make it habitable and just and humane. Noting that causality exists in nature does not permit us to defer to moral laws that govern nature, or we would not have a moral warrant to give protease inhibitors to persons with AIDS or use vaccination to eliminate smallpox. This is a fundamental distinction and one that we need to address rationally. Intervention in nature is not "tinkering," meaning a frivolous, foolish activity. Our alteration of nature is a serious act and, frankly, a violent act that is always understood to be one of power, a power that must be contained. There is no intervention in nature that is not an example of disciplined violence—not cooking food with flames and knives, or raising chickens in a world of raccoons, or growing tomatoes and pulling out the weeds and crushing the insects, or recombining DNA to make monoclonal antibodies. To think otherwise is to live in Disneyland, with a fantasy self-image as a noble savage, a romantic served by invisible hands. The point of stewardship is not passivity, but the complex task of intervention, prudence, and hard work. Leaving the natural world alone has never been a part of the human response, because we believe in the protection of the vulnerable and we believe in justice. Act as I do, says God in the biblical texts. Live as God does, say the prophets of many faiths. Transform the world and see beyond your animal horizon.

Learning and Studying

We are readers of text. As moral actors, we are enjoined to learn the text, to read carefully and to study what we see. Let me extrapolate. Learning and study of the text of the law, and of philosophy and humanities, and reading the texts of the phenomenological world, is the task of humans. We are curious to understand. Like Bacon, Franklin, and Darwin, we like to observe to "read" and then write of the word and the world. For research into such new terrain as stem cells, we can understand our drive toward interpretation in several ways. First, we can understand the power the essential human narrative has for us, recognizing that it is a story that has been deconstructed by a different reading of nature in the last century. Adam and Eve, marriage and love, heterosexual procreative union and the production and rearing of one's biological child—these are not such a simple matter in contemporary times, even for conservative thinkers. We have first come to understand gametes, and then the way that genes are arranged in each gamete, and the way that sperm and egg can be artificially taken from the bodies of people, mixed, implanted in surrogate mothers, raised by still others, all of whom we are prepared to call loving parents. The story of human birth can have many beginnings. Now we see that the fate of blastocysts can be also understood as having different endings—a blastocyst may be successfully implanted in a human womb or it may fail to implant, as most of them do. It may be frozen until it decomposes, as perhaps more than 100,000 of them are doing now. Or it may be used to make stem cells. Once we have taken a gamete from a body, and once we have mixed it outside a body, any artificial fate is equally experimental, equally artifact. At any point in any of this—from in vitro fertilization to stem cell production—the fabricated embryo may be destroyed. We read the plot line into the phenomena—we as readers give it shape and structure. The blastocyst is flat at the five-day stage. It is organized only if a gene activates correctly, which is an event influenced by internal and external factors. (Think here of a sheet of paper in your hands—it can be folded into various things—a fortune teller game, a paper airplane, or a hat—at what point do we name this as its potential, as the thing itself?)

Much of the world that we seek to read is not revealed to us. This is a fundamental truth of the human condition, that we live in a world not only unfinished, unredeemed, but not yet understood. Part of the task of the scientific method is to support radical awe with careful experimentation, with hypothesis and guesswork, and after experiments, then retesting and rereading data. The real way that science works is by hunches, by learning to see, know, and understand the way the world works long before it can be altered. Despite claims made about cures, or claims made about monsters made in the lab, real-life biology is far from cures. Stem cells may lead to tissue transplants, and then again they may not. Who can really know yet? And that is precisely the point. What stem cell and genetic research can do right now is help us learn about far more basic things, such as how parts of cells signal to other parts, how proteins are made, why cells die and why they grow. Unless the slow guesswork and chance of science is permitted, we never will get to the human medical trials at all. Basic science is a kind of free reading of newly found scrolls. It would be tragic if we cannot read them with freedom, allowing the hypothesis to be tested, allowing the first and second and then many more of our tries to be wrong. That we do not know the future is the whole point of science. It is not some aberration to be feared.

This is a theological point, but it is one that, as a moral philosopher, I am led to make. It is perhaps the case that we are led to this moment of understanding precisely to learn about the mutability and plasticity of the world, down to our very cells. Perhaps it is given to us to be able to decode and decipher this particular mystery at this particular time. For Jews, the world calls out to be read, as a text is said to call out, "Interpret me!" In this place, we have the possibility to understand creation—of families, of fates, and of the remarkable language of DNA—differently, that we have a beginner's sense of reading fully.

This postmodern philosophical idea that all narrative acts are acts of interpretation, with many causes and many versions, and that the world is far more changeable than we think is actually a very old idea. Indeed, it is the premise behind the way the Jews, Muslims, and Christians thought about magic. The idea of magic as a metaphor for stem cell research, and in particular the kind of magic that alchemy was for the ancients, is a useful one. Magic enters into our debate because the scientists themselves speak of stem cells as "magic," and, like alchemy, the research is predicated on understanding how small units—in our case cells, and in their case base metals—can combine into complex and valuable matter. The alchemists yearned for magic that would turn the ordinary into gold, and were also seeking immortality for instance in the sorcerer's stone, and both pursuits are familiar to us. That the use of magic was actual and achievable and valid under some circumstances did not render it harmless. Indeed, the power of creation was wielded by the recombination of the letters of God's name. In talmudic texts, the trick of magical creation was the trick of reading correctly.

In considering how to best use magical authority, the rabbinic community set limits on its use. In a long and complex debate, they come to agree that it is proper to make even living entities with the use of words and incantation, but they must be made within limits, for a tangible and useful and serious purpose, within the cultural norms and without violation, and only in the company of others as a part of careful study. But the debate ends with a clear support for the act of reading and writing things into being. All such study, even magic, is permitted in order to learn. Permission to do the action is a separate matter, but there is no magic that we are not permitted to study. "All must be learned in order to teach." To teach, as Bob Gibbs notes, is to be asked questions, to be interrupted in telling by disruptive questions, and hence to be able to learn to teach warrants basic research as a part of a social society.

Solidarity and Community

We have a duty to be relational, in solidarity and community with others. Moral status is related to temporality, moral location, and relationships of power. The argument from Jewish and Islamic and many Protestants and secular sources is not that embryos do not matter, but that they are developing toward full membership in our social contract. Humans are born into this duty. One of the ways we experience the self is in the eyes of the other, and hence, as we are bound into duty for the other, she is bound into duty to us. Social contracts require the fact of our primary relationality for states to be held together. It is a premise of such contracts that not all choices will be ful-filled, but that states are held together by mutual regard, human flourishing. In thinking about stem cell research, the demand for social solidarity means we must be attentive to the process of how such cells are created and how eggs are collected from the bodies of women. To replicate the most ex-ploitative aspects of the fertility clinic would undermine the premise of a mu-tually obligated community.

Principles of ethics have emerged from many different places and theories of morality. The six moral duties I have suggested are not ones that we agree on now, but I would suggest that they are based on good arguments. Such duties are both normative and descriptive, for in telling us who we might be and what we might do, they both limit and free us.

ELEVEN

Talking Like Believers: Christians and Jews in the Embryonic Stem Cell Debate

SONDRA WHEELER

The first requirement for religious communities who want to reckon seriously with the ethical questions raised by the use of embryonic stem cells in research (ESCR) is to get their facts straight. This means they have to learn enough about the biology of reproduction, and about the actual characteristics and developmental trajectory of these very early embryos, to be clear about what they are dealing with. This involves understanding the basic structure of the entities under discussion, including such things as the kind of organization and degree of cellular differentiation present in the early embryo and blastocyst at various points in their development.

For instance, a five-day-old blastocyst has approximately 64–128 cells. It is divided into an inner cell mass of pluripotent cells (all identical to one another) and a trophoblast, a layer of likewise identical outer cells that enables the blastocyst to implant in the uterine wall. This will become the placenta if development proceeds normally. Details of this kind are critical, both for what they tell us positively and for what they rule out. For example, it is not the case that the embryonic stem cells themselves are the equivalent of an embryo. Lacking the means to form a placenta, they cannot implant and develop independently. What is problematic for many is that what one has to do to obtain these stem cells is to disaggregate what clearly is an embryo, which all acknowledge might be capable of developing into a person.

Getting our information straight also includes understanding something of the biological programming that directs these early embryos toward the successive stages of their existence. This programming is given in the DNA complete at fertilization (or at the time of cellular fusion in the case of an embryo formed by somatic cell nuclear transfer, or SCNTC). It is the genetic connection to the biological parents (or the replication of a single human nucleus donor in SCNTC) as well as the genetically directed character of human development that causes some people to regard this very primitive form of human life as, morally speaking, "one of us." Under ordinary circumstances, the early embryo is a genetically unique, self-directing, and self-regulating living entity that will, if all goes well, develop into a fetus and be born an infant to whom we will automatically ascribe full human status. It is on this ground that some people regard even early embryos as entitled to protection as a being whose origin and destiny both connect it to the broader human community.

But paying attention to the actual character of the beings under discussion further requires that we understand how they fit into their context as part of the living system of the body, and all the various contingencies that determine whether a given embryo continues to develop, is implanted, comes to term, and is delivered some thirty-eight weeks later. We must take note of all the natural uncertainties that attend the existence of this very early form of human life, such that it seems that fewer than half of fertilized embryos successfully survive to implant and begin development. In addition, it is rare but possible in early stages for two embryos to fuse into a single embryo and develop into one normal individual or, conversely, for a single embryo to split into two embryos that develop into two genetically identical but fully distinct human beings. All these facts complicate the readiness to regard a very early embryo as already entitled to the full protection granted a human being, when its continued development and individuality are yet so uncertain.

This careful attention to the facts is essential because, at least among theistic traditions, the encounter with material reality is here and everywhere the encounter with creation, and thus with the creative intention of God. One broad and deep strand of Jewish and Christian thought draws on this identification as well as on a notion of the "fittedness" of human perception and reason to discern something of the divine intention from the character and ordering of the world we encounter. One need not be a natural law theologian of full-blown Scholastic commitments to recognize that part of how we discern what is due in justice to a being is to attend to the reality of that being: its origin, its characteristics and capacities, and the foreseeable path along which its existence moves. Paying attention to what can be known of the world is part of how we honor God's creation, both in the objects of our attention and in ourselves. As rational creatures, we "participate" in God's ordering of the world by seeing, knowing, and loving that order. Human understanding is in itself an act of praise and obedience in which we embrace our distinctive character as images of God.

Having said all this, it is still important to have a realistic and chastened view of what such attention will and will not provide us. We cannot go looking for "moral status" or "value" as if it were a feature we might locate under a microscope if only we had one powerful enough. Even if our knowledge of moral standing is partly derived from the facts and character of existence, it remains a distinct, second-order judgment. That is, it is something we construct in response to what we see and not something we read off as a characteristic like color or mass or chemical composition. There is no way to get ourselves off the hook of making a kind of judgment about the moral standing of the early embryo as part of our judgment of the ethics of ESCR. A sound understanding of the characteristics, natural history, and normal development of that embryo must inform that judgment, but it will never render it unnecessary.

How We Talk and Why It Matters

One of the things that must characterize discussions of the ethics of ESCR among communities of Jewish and Christian faith is an exemplary (and sorely needed) care about the language with which we make our observations, frame our questions, and characterize our findings. Such care is always both an intellectual and a moral obligation in ethical discourse, but it takes on particular importance in the present controversy. In this highly charged debate, there are a number of stakeholders in the public conversation about ESCR, people and groups who come to it with a particular point of view or a particular conclusion to articulate and defend. These include those who have a share in the research itself and thus have a professional stake in the pursuit of particular lines of inquiry. It also includes those who face diseases in themselves or in their loved ones for which this research is thought to hold some future hope of benefit. It includes likewise those who have settled moral positions on other issues, which impinge on the status of early human life in one direction or the other, and so are driven by consistency either to support or to oppose ESCR. Finally, it includes representatives of (and professional spokespersons for) the various scientific and commercial entities that have great human and material resources invested in present or projected research and a consequent personal and economic stake in the outcome. These people are operating out of diverse and ultimately unknowable motives. Without attributing any ill will or intentional deception to them, it is easy to see the way in which these interests and commitments shape the language in which ostensibly neutral information is conveyed.

Here I am not thinking of the more obvious and extreme cases in which those who oppose using embryonic stem cells characterize their adversaries as advocating the wanton killing of the unborn, while proponents speak of those who care more for blastocysts than for living, suffering human beings. I am thinking of the more subtle judgments enfolded in what purports to be descriptive language. For example, those who fear the engineering possibilities afforded by ESCR allied to embryo cloning raise the fears of others by speaking of stem cell research as leading directly to "designer babies." Those who hope for future therapies that might be developed from these avenues of research speak about the target maladies as "scourges" about to be eradicated, language that recalls the great plagues. It reinforces the impression that we face an overwhelming threat, in the face of which moral qualms about the destruction of embryos must be put aside in favor of immediate action to stave off disaster. Neither characterization of the results to be expected from research on embryonic stem cells is fair or accurate.

Also to be eschewed are formations that misstate or misrepresent what the ethical questions actually are in favor of questions that are either easier to answer or more rhetorically exciting. Examples include asking whether the embryo is alive, something that, speaking purely biologically, cannot be doubted (if it were not, it could not provide living and replicating embryonic stem cells). On the other end of the spectrum is construing the issue to be whether a five-day-old embryo is the same as a fully formed and functioning human being, which it obviously is not. The question is this: is a human embryo a kind of thing that we may intentionally destroy, or even create in a laboratory with the advance intention of destroying it? To do so is to make the embryo unequivocally a means to an end in which it has no part. Many of those who would not regard the embryo's claim to protection as morally comparable to that of a human being at later stages of development nonetheless reject such a complete instrumentalization of a form of human life, however rudimentary.

In this controversy, as in all moral debates of importance, the reality at stake is complex and ambiguous, and moral judgment about how we ought to respond to it is genuinely difficult. If our aim is bearing public witness to moral truth, on the one hand, and the formation and protection of the conscience of believers, on the other, we will speak with care and test the content and tone of all our speech by the norm of what advances the truth and sustains a conversation whose aim is wise discernment. To do otherwise is not only to obscure the question at hand, but to fray the ties of respect and trust that enable our churches and synagogues to be contexts for moral discernment and moral accountability in the first place. What we thereby place at risk is more important than our winning or losing a particular moral argument; it is our identity and viability as communities of faith.

Doing Ethics for Planet Earth

One of the greatest challenges in doing social ethics is paying close and serious attention to the actual contexts in which questions arise and are pursued, which are also the contexts in which whatever answers we propose will take their effect. It is always tempting to work out a moral position simply by applying general commitments grounded in religious principles or secular moral theory to a new set of questions. But to do so is to attend to the rational consistency of our moral models at the expense of realism and sensitivity about the landscape within which moral judgments are actually lived out.

The current debate about the ethics of ESCR is a particularly vivid example of such myopia, because it tends to address the question of ESCR quite as if the embryos we contemplate using as source material had suddenly been off-loaded from space ships. In reality, of course, the possibility and the question of ESCR arises only because of a number of earlier steps we have taken as a society, with more or (often) less reflection, debate, and deliberation. It is the rapidly growing, unregulated, and largely uninspected reproductive technology industry that produced these so-called leftover embryos, frequently under conditions that raise both ethical and scientific questions about their use. They are simply what is left behind by the in vitro fertilization technology whose use we have come to take for granted in the last two decades.

But whether we decide we ought to use these embryos for research or refrain from doing so, the questions they raise for us all will not go away. While we are arguing about what we may do with the estimated 100,000–200,000 embryos currently in frozen storage in this country alone, we expect to make another 20,000 per year for the foreseeable future. If the prospect of actively destroying them by disaggregation for the sake of potential therapeutic benefits is troubling, then we have a number of other problems to resolve. For how can we flinch from deliberate destruction if we are unperturbed by wholesale discard or by cold storage lasting so long that whatever potential viability these embryos may have had is lost? If we are at all consistent in our moral thinking, our struggle over the status of early embryos will have profound and perhaps dramatic implications for how we think, talk, and behave regarding reproductive technologies in general. Communities of faith have an enormous stake in these matters, for they have powerful implications for the moral meaning of our embodied procreative power, and they significantly affect how we understand the relationship between the generations.

We must also bear in mind the social and economic framework within which this research is taking place. This involves some clear-eyed realism about the resources and motives that lie behind its development and what will shape the selection, development, and distribution of any clinical advances or medical products that arise from it. Before we are swayed by those who wax rhapsodic about the unlimited potential for curing Parkinson's or repairing devastating spinal cord injuries, we do well to remember the role of marketability in determining what products do and do not get made by pharmaceutical companies that are and remain profit-making enterprises. We need to pay attention to who does and who does not receive the cutting-edge drugs and therapies presently available. In view of the fact that all Americans do not yet have access to even basic preventive medicine or the first-line treatments of primary care, it is disingenuous to weigh the potential benefits of ESCR as if the barriers to access to advanced therapies are about to dissolve. We already have a wide range of drugs and treatment protocols for life-threatening illnesses that are available only to those who can pay or whose insurance is sufficiently comprehensive. It is sobering to remember that the high-powered techniques of assisted reproduction that brought these disputed embryos into existence remain available only to a very small fraction of those who face infertility.

More broadly, we must attend to, analyze, and challenge the cultural context that permeates this and all conversations about right and wrong in the development and application of new biotechnology. Ours is a culture in which expediency is the moral coin of the realm. Even conversations that purport to be about matters of principle soon give way to utilitarian calculations, as we entertain projections of just how useful it will be if we decide that no countervailing duty offers a barrier to our projects. In this regard, it is illuminating to note the recent shift in public conversation about the moral permissibility of various uses of early embryos for research. For many months, the dominant position among supporters of ESCR was that it would be morally tolerable to use existing embryos left over from fertility clinics that were otherwise slated for discard, but not to create embryos in the laboratory solely for research purposes. More recently, as a professional lobbyist remarked, the topic in regulatory contexts has been "all cloning, all the time," as the desirability of creating cloned embryos by SCNTC as a source of genetically matched stem cells has become more evident. (This is the source of the present resistance to a proposed Senate ban on human cloning, worded in such a way as to rule out not only reproductive cloning but research-related cloning as well.) Without arguing a position either way, it is important to note that such a protocol would involve precisely the creation of embryos in laboratories for research purposes. What is significant is the largely unheralded shift in the moral ground of the conversation and how quickly it has come about. Clearly, whatever guidelines or rules about the use of human embryos in research we put in place will be subject to review and revision before the ink is dry, and what once seemed to be bright lines have a way of fading into obscurity.

As a final element of attention to context, religious communities must retain their critical distance from and critical perspective on the culture in which they are embedded and by which they are so often compromised and coopted. Ours is a society that is enormously productive and remarkably efficient and adaptable in the creation and distribution of material goods to supply our needs and desires. It is also a society in which the body alive or dead is relentlessly commodified, valued as tissue source and container of genetic information, over and above the ancient objectification of body-as-laborer. As we extend the pursuit of happiness as far as our resources and ingenuity will take us, shaped by the goals of freedom from suffering of every kind and the provision of whatever will make us happy, increasing alienation from our bodily existence is the price we pay for the exaltation of the will and the evasion of every bodily limitation. This is the overarching context within which all our reflection and thinking about bioethics takes place. To fail to take it seriously is to deceive ourselves and render our conversation largely irrelevant to the reality we seek to shape.

Speaking Our Own Languages

Above everything else, communities of faith must address these questions as confessional communities, as those who are not just characterized but constituted by fundamental theological convictions about the source and aims and end of human existence. Churches and synagogues can and must speak not as ersatz public policy engineers, but as genuine theological communities, out of and not incidental to their own identity. This means returning ever and again to the basic elements of our professions of faith. These include, as noted earlier, a doctrine of creation, which receives the world not as happenstance nor as machine but as gift, an expression of the will and character of God. Christians and Jews share as well a theology of providence, the conviction that God has not abandoned the world God has made but continues to be engaged with it as Sustainer and Judge and Redeemer. Belief in the providence of God need not take the naive and implausible form demolished by Enlightenment skepticism, a form that could acknowledge neither mystery nor tragedy in the course of life. Such a view was never part of biblical faith to begin with. What is and has always been essential to both traditions is a fundamental conviction that God is God indeed, and worthy of trust. It is not a denial of pain, but a confidence in redemption, that distinguishes faith from unbelief.

What arises from this web of convictions is a theological anthropology, a distinctive account of the nature and purpose and meaning of human life. It is an account that does not see the fullness of life finally in terms of the avoidance of suffering or the successful overcoming of the vulnerability and contingency of mortal existence. According to this view, the meaning of life is rather to be found in the depth and fidelity of relationships. Christians and Jews assert that, in its most fundamental form, the meaning of life is that we are to love God with all our heart and soul and mind and strength and our neighbors as ourselves. Within the biblical witness that is the foundation of both communities, it is to a great extent taken for granted that the cost of fidelity in a world marred by sin will sometimes entail suffering. Such suffering is viewed without romanticism—it is a genuine evil—but also without terror, for God is greater than suffering and can and will comfort and redeem us beyond all hope.

The implications of such convictions for questions of the legitimate aims and methods of medicine, and the appropriate avenues of research, may not be immediately evident. Nonetheless, they are fundamental. For such an anthropology tells us what we are to strive for first and last, and what are the ultimate goals that both undergird and limit the ends we seek in all our more proximate undertakings. The love of God and neighbor that impels us at once affirms the pursuit of health and the amelioration of suffering (for God's will is for flourishing) and constrains what we may do in service of those ends.

The acknowledged aims of medicine are to prevent, to heal, or to alleviate the effects of disease and bodily dysfunction, and these are well and good. But clearly these aims are not ultimate. Not only are they decisively limited by the mortality of the body, but they are pursued not simply in themselves but for the sake of the fullness of human life and love that they make possible.

As we consider what we may and what we ought to do in search of therapies to mitigate or overcome the effects of injury, aging, and illness, we cannot base our moral judgments solely on the goodness of the outcomes we hope to achieve in our research. It is essential that we also pay attention to the means we adopt to secure those outcomes. We need all the honesty, care, and objectivity we can muster as we contemplate both the sort of beings we make use of in research involving the creation and destruction of human embryos and the sort of beings we become in doing so. Questions about the ethics of ESCR must be entertained for what they are, part of larger questions about who we are and where our good lies and how it is to be pursued. The essential attribute of communities of faith is that they insist on placing all particular questions in the context of these overarching questions, answers to which are the peculiar terrain of theology. This insistence is their vocation and their unique contribution to the public debate about biotechnology and the ethics of research.

Appendices

Declaration on the Production and the Scientific and Therapeutic Use of Human Embryonic Stem Cells

PONTIFICAL ACADEMY FOR LIFE

This document seeks to contribute to the debate on the production and use of embryonic stem cells which is now taking place in scientific and ethical literature and in public opinion. Given the growing relevance of the debate on the limits and licity of the production and use of such cells, there is a pressing need to reflect on the ethical implications which are present.

The first section will very briefly set out the most recent scientific data on stem cells and the biotechnological data on their production and use. The second section will draw attention to the more relevant ethical problems raised by these new discoveries and their applications.

Scientific Aspects

Although some aspects need to be studied more thoroughly, a commonly accepted definition of "stem cell" describes it as a cell with two characteristics: 1) the property of an unlimited self-maintenance—that is, the ability to reproduce itself over a long period of time without becoming differentiated; and 2) the capability to produce non-permanent progenitor cells, with limited capacity for proliferation, from which derive a variety of lineages of highly differentiated cells (neural cells, muscle cells, blood cells, etc.). For about thirty years stem cells have provided a vast field of research in adult tissue,[1] in embryonic tissue and in in vitro cultures of embryonic stem cells of experimental animals.[2] But public attention has recently increased with a new milestone that has been reached: the production of human embryonic stem cells.

Human Embryonic Stem Cells

Today, the preparation of human embryonic stem cells (human ES cells) implies the following:[3] 1) the production of human embryos and/or the use of the surplus embryos resulting from in vitro fertilization or of frozen embryos; 2) the development of these embryos to the stage of initial blastocysts; 3) the isolation of the embryoblast or inner cell mass (ICM)—which implies the destruction of the embryo; 4) culturing these cells on a feeder layer of irradiated mouse embryonic fibroblasts in a suitable medium, where they can multiply and coalesce to form colonies; 5) repeated subculturing of these colonies, which lead to the formation of cell lines capable of multiplying indefinitely while preserving the characteristics of ES cells for months and years.

These ES cells, however, are only the point of departure for the preparation of differentiated cell lines, that is, of cells with the characteristics proper of the various tissues (muscle, neural, epithelial, haematic, germinal, etc.). Methods for obtaining them are still being studied;[4] but the injection of human ES cells into experimental animals (mice) or their culture in vitro in controlled environments to their confluence have shown that they are able to produce differentiated cells which, in a normal development, would derive from the three different embryonic tissue layers: endoderm (intestinal epithelium), mesoderm (cartilage, bone, smooth and striated muscle) and ectoderm (neural epithelium, squamous epithelium).[5]

The results of these experiments had a great impact on the world of both science and biotechnology—especially medicine and pharmacology—no less than the world of business and the mass media. There were high hopes that the application of this knowledge would lead to new and safer ways of treating serious diseases, something which had been sought for years.[6] But the impact was greatest in the political world.[7] In the United States in particular, in response to the long-standing opposition of Congress to the use of federal funds for research in which human embryos were destroyed, there came strong pressure from the National Institutes of Health (NIH), among others, to obtain funds for at least using stem cells produced by private groups; there came also recommendations from the National Bioethics Advisory Committee (NBAC), established by the Federal Government to study the problem, that public money should be given not only for research on embryonic stem cells but also for producing them. Indeed, persistent efforts are being made to rescind definitively the present legal ban on the use of federal funds for research on human embryos. Similar pressures are being brought to bear also in England, Japan and Australia.

Therapeutic Cloning

It had become clear that the therapeutic use of ES cells, as such, entailed significant risks, since—as had been observed in experiments on mice—tumours resulted. It would have been necessary therefore to prepare specialized lines of differentiated cells as they were needed; and it did not appear that this could be done in a short period of time. But, even if successful, it would have been very difficult to be certain that the inoculation or therapeutic implant was free of stem cells, which would entail the corresponding risks. Moreover there would have been a need for further treatment to overcome immunological incompatibility. For these reasons, three methods of therapeutic cloning[8] were proposed, suitable for preparing pluripotent human embryonic stem cells with well defined genetic information from which desired differentiation would then follow.

1. The replacement of the nucleus of an oocyte with the nucleus of an adult cell of a given subject, followed by embryonic development to the stage of blastocyst and the use of the inner cell mass (ICM) in order to obtain ES cells and, from these, the desired differentiated cells.
2. The transfer of a nucleus of a cell of a given subject into an oocite of another animal. An eventual success in this procedure should lead—it is presumed—to the development of a human embryo, to be used as in the preceding case.
3. The reprogramming of the nucleus of a cell of a given subject by fusing the ES cytoplast with a somatic cell karyoplast, thus obtaining a "cybrid." This is a possibility which is still under study. In any event, this method too would seem to demand a prior preparation of ES cells from human embryos.

Current scientific research is looking to the first of these possibilities as the preferred method, but it is obvious that—from a moral point of view, as we shall see—all three proposed solutions are unacceptable.

Adult Stem Cells

From studies on adult stem cells (ASC) in the last thirty years it had been clearly shown that many adult tissues contain stem cells, but stem cells capable of producing only cells proper to a given tissue. That is, it was not thought that these cells could be reprogrammed. In more recent years,[9] however, pluripotent stem cells were also discovered in various human tissues—in bone marrow (HSCs), in the brain (NSCs), in the mesenchyme (MSCs) of various organs, and in umbilical cord blood (P/CB, placental/cord blood); these are cells capable of producing different types of cells, mostly blood cells, muscle cells and neural cells. It was learnt how to recognize them, select them, maintain them in development, and induce them to form different types of mature cells by means of growth factors and other regulating proteins. Indeed noteworthy progress has already been made in the experimental field, applying the most advanced methods of genetic engineering and molecular biology in analyzing the genetic programme at work in stem cells,[10] and in importing the desired genes into stem cells or progenitor cells which, when implanted, are able to restore specific functions to damaged tissue.[11] It is sufficient to mention, on the basis of the reported references, that in human beings the stem cells of bone marrow, from which the different lines of blood cells are formed, have as their marker the molecule CD34; and that, when purified, these cells are able to restore entirely the normal blood count in patients who receive ablative doses of radiation and chemotherapy, and this with a speed which is in proportion to the quantity of cells used. Furthermore, there are already indications on how to guide the development of neural stem cells (NSCs) through the use of various proteins—among them neuroregulin and bone morphogenetic protein 2 (BMP2)—which can direct NSCs to become neurons or glia (myelin-producing neural support cells) or even smooth muscle tissue.

The note of satisfaction, albeit cautious, with which many of the cited works conclude is an indication of the great promise that "adult stem cells" offer for effective treatment of many pathologies. Thus the affirmation made by D. J. Watt and G. E. Jones: "The muscle stem cell, whether it be of the embryonic myoblast lineage, or of the adult satellite status, may well turn out to be a cell with far greater importance to tissues other than its tissue of origin and may well hold the key to future therapies for diseases other than those of a myogenic nature" (p. 93). As J. A. Nolta and D. B. Kohn emphasize: "Progress in the use of gene transfer into haemotopoietic cells has led to initial clinical trials. Information developed by these early efforts will be used to guide future developments. Ultimately, gene therapy may allow a number of genetic and acquired diseases to be treated, without the current complications from bone marrow transplantation with allogeneic cells" (p. 460); and the confirmation offered by D. L. Clarke and J. Frisén: "These studies suggest that stem cells in different adult tissues may be more similar than previously thought and perhaps in some cases have a developmental repertoire close to that of ES cells" (p. 1663) and "demonstrates that an adult neural stem cell has a very broad developmental capacity and may potentially be used to generate a variety of cell types for transplantation in different diseases" (p. 1660).

The progress and results obtained in the field of adult stem cells (ASC) show not only their great plasticity but also their many possible uses, in all likelihood no different from those of embryonic stem cells, since plasticity depends in large part upon genetic information, which can be reprogrammed.

Obviously, it is not yet possible to compare the therapeutic results obtained and obtainable using embryonic stem cells and adult stem cells. For the latter, various pharmaceutical firms are already conducting clinical experiments[12] which are showing success and raising genuine hopes for the not too distant future. With embryonic stem cells, even if various experimental approaches prove positive,[13] their application in the clinical field—owing precisely to the serious ethical and legal problems which arise—needs to be seriously reconsidered and requires a great sense of responsibility before the dignity of every human being.

Ethical Problems

Given the nature of this article, the key ethical problems implied by these new technologies are presented briefly, with an indication of the responses which emerge from a careful consideration of the human subject from the moment of conception. It is this consideration which underlies the position affirmed and put forth by the Magisterium of the Church.

The first ethical problem, which is fundamental, can be formulated thus: Is it morally licit to produce and/or use living human embryos for the preparation of ES cells?

The answer is negative, for the following reasons:

1. On the basis of a complete biological analysis, the living human embryo is—from the moment of the union of the gametes—a human subject with a well defined identity, which from that point begins its own coordinated, continuous and gradual development, such that at no later stage can it be considered as a simple mass of cells.[14]
2. From this it follows that as a "human individual" it has the right to its own life; and therefore every intervention which is not in favour of the embryo is an act which violates that right. Moral theology has always

taught that in the case of "jus certum tertii" the system of probabilism does not apply.[15]

3. Therefore, the ablation of the inner cell mass (ICM) of the blastocyst, which critically and irremediably damages the human embryo, curtailing its development, is a gravely immoral act and consequently is gravely illicit.

4. No end believed to be good, such as the use of stem cells for the preparation of other differentiated cells to be used in what look to be promising therapeutic procedures, can justify an intervention of this kind. A good end does not make right an action which in itself is wrong.

5. For Catholics, this position is explicitly confirmed by the Magisterium of the Church which, in the Encyclical Evangelium Vitae, with reference to the Instruction Donum Vitae of the Congregation for the Doctrine of the Faith, affirms: "The Church has always taught and continues to teach that the result of human procreation, from the first moment of its existence, must be guaranteed that unconditional respect which is morally due to the human being in his or her totality and unity in body and spirit: 'The human being is to be respected and treated as a person from the moment of conception; and therefore from that same moment his rights as a person must be recognized, among which in the first place is the inviolable right of every innocent human being to life'" (No. 60).[16]

The second ethical problem can be formulated thus: Is it morally licit to engage in so-called "therapeutic cloning" by producing cloned human embryos and then destroying them in order to produce ES cells?

The answer is negative, for the following reason: Every type of therapeutic cloning, which implies producing human embryos and then destroying them in order to obtain stem cells, is illicit; for there is present the ethical problem examined above, which can only be answered in the negative.[17]

The third ethical problem can be formulated thus: Is it morally licit to use ES cells, and the differentiated cells obtained from them, which are supplied by other researchers or are commercially obtainable?

The answer is negative, since: prescinding from the participation—formal or otherwise—in the morally illicit intention of the principal agent, the case in question entails a proximate material cooperation in the production and manipulation of human embryos on the part of those producing or supplying them. In conclusion, it is not hard to see the seriousness and gravity of the ethical problem posed by the desire to extend to the field of human research the production and/or use of human embryos, even from an humanitarian perspective. The possibility, now confirmed, of using adult stem cells to attain the same goals as would be sought with embryonic stem cells—even if many further steps in both areas are necessary before clear and conclusive results are obtained—indicates that adult stem cells represent a more reasonable and human method for making correct and sound progress in this new field of research and in the therapeutic applications which it promises. These applications are undoubtedly a source of great hope for a significant number of suffering people.

The President
Prof. Juan de Dios Vial Correa
The Vice President
S.E. Mons. Elio Sgreccia
Vatican City, August 25, 2000.

Notes

1. Cf. M. Loeffler, C. S. Potten, "Stem Cells and Cellular Pedigrees—a Conceptual Introduction" in C. S. Potten (ed.), *Stem Cells,* Academic Press, London (1997), pp. 1–27; D. Van der Kooy, S. Weiss, "Why Stem Cells?" *Science* 2000, 287, 1439–1441.

2. Cf. T. Nakano, H. Kodama, T. Honjo, Generation of Lymphohematopoietic Cells from Embryonic Stem Cells in Culture," *Science* 1994, 265, 1098–1101; G. Keller, "In Vitro Differentiation of Embryonic Stem Cells," *Current Opinion in Cell Biology* 1995, 7 862–869; S. Robertson, M. Kennedy, G. Keller, "Hematopoietic Commitment During Embryogenesis," *Annals of the New York Academy of Sciences* 1999, 872, 9–16.

3. Cf. J. A. Thomson, J. Itskovitz-Eldor, S. S. Shapiro, et al., "Embryonic Stem Cell Lines Derived from Human Blastocysts," *Science* 1998, 282, 1145–1147; G. Vogel, "Harnessing the Power of Stem Cells," *Science* 1999, 183, 1432–1434.

4. Cf. F. M. Watt, B. L. M. Hogan, "Out of Eden: Stem Cells and Their Niches," *Science* 2000, 287, 1427–1430.

5. Cf. J. A. Thomson, J. Itskovitz-Eldor, S. S. Shapiro et al., op. cit.

6. Cf. U. S. Congress, Office of Technology Assessment, "Neural Grafting: Repairing the Brain and Spinal Cord," OTA-BA-462, Washington, DC, US Government Printing Office, 1990; A. McLaren, "Stem Cells: Golden Opportunities with Ethical Baggage," *Science* 2000, 288, 1778.

7. Cf. E. Marshall, "A Versatile Cell Line Raises Scientific Hopes, Legal Questions," *Science* 1998, 282, 1014–1015; J. Gearhart, "New Potential for Human Embryonic Stem Cells," ibid., 1061–1062; E. Marshall, "Britain Urged to Expand Embryo Studies," ibid., 216–2168; 73 *Scientists,* "Science over Politics," *Science* 1999, 283, 1849–1850; E. Marshall, "Ethicists Back Stem Cell Research, White House Treads Cautiously," *Science* 1999, 285,

502; H. T. Shapiro, "Ethical Dilemmas and Stem Cell Research," ibid., 2065; G. Vogel, "NIH Sets Rules for Funding Embryonic Stem Cell Research," *Science* 1999, 286, 2050; G. Keller, H. R. Snodgrass, "Human Embryonic Stem Cells: The Future Is Now," *Nature Medicine* 1999, 5, 151–152; G. J. Annas, A. Caplan, S. Elias, "Stem Cell Politics, Ethics and Medical Progress," ibid., 1339–1341; G. Vogel, "Company Gets Rights to Cloned Human Embryos," *Science* 2000, 287, 559; D. Normile, "Report Would Open Up Research in Japan," ibid., 949; M. S. Frankel, "In Search of Stem Cell Policy," ibid., 1397; D. Perry, "Patients Voices: The Powerful Sound in the Stem Cell Debate," ibid., 1423; N. Lenoir, "Europe Confronts the Embryonic Stem Cell Research Challenge," ibid., 1425–1427; F. E. Young, "A Time for Restraint," ibid., 1424; Editorial, "Stem Cells," *Nature Medicine* 2000, 6, 231.

8. D. Davor, J. Gearhart, "Putting Stem Cells to Work," *Science* 1999, 283, 1468–1470.

9 Cf. C. S. Potten (ed.), *Stem Cells* (London: Academic Press, 1997), p. 474; D. Orlic, T. A. Bock, L. Kanz, "Hemopoietic Stem Cells: Biology and Transplantation," *Ann. N.Y. Acad. Sciences,* vol. 872, New York 1999, p. 405; M. F. Pittenger, A. M. Mackay, S. C. Beck et al., "Multilineage Potential of Adult Human Mesenchymal Stem Cells," *Science* 1999, 284, 143–147; C. R. R. Bjornson, R. L. Rietze, B.A. Reynolds et al., "Turning Brain into Blood: A Hematopoietic Fate Adopted by Adult Neural Stem Cells in vivo," *Science* 1999, 183, 534–536; V. Ourednik, J. Ourednik, K. I. Park, E. Y. Snyder, "Neural Stem Cells—A Versatile Tool for Cell Replacement and Gene Therapy in the Central Nervous System," *Clinical Genetics* 1999, 56, 167–178; I. Lemischka, "Searching for Stem Cell Regulatory Molecules: Some General Thoughts and Possible Approaches," *Ann. N.Y.Acad. Sci.* 1999, 872, 274–288; H. H. Gage, "Mammalian Neural Stem Cells," *Science* 2000, 287, 1433–1438; D. L. Clarke, C. B. Johansson, J. Frisen et al., "Generalized Potential of Adult Neural Stem Cells," *Science* 2000, 288, 1660–1663; G. Vogel, "Brain Cells Reveal Surprising Versatility," ibid., 1559–1561.

10. Cf. R. L. Phillips, R. E. Ernst, I. R. Lemischka, et al., "The Genetic Program of Hematopoietic Stem Cells," *Science* 2000, 288, 1635–1640.

11. Cf. D. J. Watt, G. E. Jones, "Skeletal Muscle Stem Cells: Function and Potential Role in Therapy," in C. S. Potten, *Stem Cells,* op. cit., 75–98; J. A. Nolta, D. B. Kohn, "Haematopoietic Stem Cells for Gene Therapy," ibid., 447–460; Y. Reisner, E. Bachar-Lustig, H-W. Li et al., "The Role of Megadose CD34+ Progenitor Cells in the Treatment of Leukemia Patients without a Matched Donor and in Tolerance Induction for Organ Transplantation," *Ann. N.Y.Acad. Sci.* 1999, 872, 336–350; D. W. Emery, G. Stamatoyannopoulous, "Stem Cell Gene Therapy for the β-Chain Hemoglobinopathies," ibid., 94–108; M. Griffith, R. Osborne, R. Munger, "Functional Human Corneal Equivalents Constructed from Cell Lines," *Science* 1999, 286, 2169–2172; N. S. Roy, S. Wang, L. Jiang et al., "In vitro Neurogenesis by Progenitor Cells Isolated from the Adult Hippocampus," *Nature Medicine* 2000, 6, 271–277; M. Noble, "Can Neural Stem Cells Be Used as Therapeutic Vehicles in the Treatment of Brain Tumors?" ibid., 369–370; I. L. Weissman, "Translating Stem and Progenitor Cell Biology to the Clinic: Barriers and Opportunities," *Science* 2000, 287, 1442–1446; P. Serup, "Planning for Pancreatic Stem Cells," *Nature Genetics* 2000, 25, 134–135.

12. E. Marshall, "The Business of Stem Cells," *Science* 2000, 287, 1419–1421.

13. Cf. O. Brustle, K. N. Jones, R. D. Learish et al., "Embryonic Stem Cell-Derived Glial Precursors: A Source of Myelinating Transplants," *Science* 1999, 285, 754–756; J. W. McDonald, X–Z Liu, Y. Qu, et al., "Transplanted Embryonic Stem Cells Survive, Differentiate and Promote Recovery in Injured Rat Spinal Cord," *Nature Medicine* 1999, 5, 1410–1412.

14. Cf. A. Serra, R. Colombo, "Identità e Statuto dell'Embrione Umano: il Contributo della Biologia," in Pontificia Academia Pro Vita, Identità e Statuto dell'Embrione Umano, Libreria Editrice Vaticana, Città del Vaticana, 1998, 00. 106–158.

15. Cf. I. Carrasco de Paula, "Il Rispetto Dovuto all'Embrione Umano: Prospettiva Storico-Dottrinale," in ibid., pp. 9–33; R. Lucas Lucas, "Statuto Antropologico dell'Embrione Umano," in ibid., pp. 159–185; M. Cozzoli, "L'Embrione Umano: Aspetti Etico-Normativi," in ibid., pp. 237–273; L. Eusebi, "La Tutela dell1Embrione Umano: Profili Giurdici," in ibid., pp. 274–286.

16. John Paul II, Encyclical Letter "Evangelium Vitae" (25 March 1995), *Acta Apostolicae Sedis* 1995, 87, 401–522; cf. also *Congregation for the Doctrine of the Faith,* "Instruction on Respect for Human Life in Its Origins and on the Dignity of Procreation 'Donum Vitae'" (22 February 1987), *Acta Apostolicae Sedis* 1988, 80, 70–102.

17. *Congregation for the Doctrine of the Faith,* op. cit., I, no. 6; C. B. Cohen (ed.), "Special Issue: Ethics and the Cloning of Human Embryos," *Kennedy Institute of Ethics Journal* 1994, n. 4, 187–282; H. T. Shapiro, "Ethical and Policy Issues of Human Cloning," *Science* 1997, 277, 195–196; M. L. Di Pietro, "Dalla Clonazione Animale all Clonazione dell'Uomo?" *Medicina el Morale* 1997, no. 6, 1099-2005; A. Serra, "Verso la Clonazione dell'Uomo? Una Nuova Frontiera della Scienza," *La Civiltà Cattolica* 1998 I, 224–234; ibid. "La Clonazione Umana in Prospettiva "Sapienziale," ibid., 329–339.

Embryonic Stem Cell Research in the Perspective of Orthodox Christianity: A Statement of the Holy Synod of Bishops of the Orthodox Church in America

Dearly-beloved in the Lord:

The current debate over research on embryonic stem cells raises in the starkest way a crucial moral question concerning the ultimate meaning and value of human life.

From the perspective of Orthodox Christianity, human life begins at conception (meaning fertilization with creation of the single-cell zygote). This conviction is grounded in the Biblical witness (e.g., Ps 139:13–16; Isaiah 49:1ff; Luke 1:41,44), as well as in the scientifically established fact that from conception there exists genetic uniqueness and cellular differentiation that, if the conceptus is allowed to develop normally, will produce a live human being.[1] Human life is sacred from its very beginning, since from conception it is ensouled existence. As such, it is "personal" existence, created in the image of God and endowed with a sanctity that destines it for eternal life.

Conservative, pro-life voices throughout the country have enthusiastically praised President Bush's recent decision regarding scientific research using human embryonic stem cells (ESCR). That decision would allow research on some sixty lines of existing stem cells, developed from human embryos which were destroyed as the cells were harvested. It would prohibit creation of embryos for research purposes, and it urges further study into the feasibility of utilizing adult stem cells to achieve the same therapeutic ends envisioned for embryonic stem cells. These limitations, it is argued, would ensure that extra embryos resulting from in vitro fertilization techniques would not be subjected to manipulation by researchers, nor would embryos be created, by cloning or any other means, for the specific purpose of serving as research subjects.

We, the Bishops of the Orthodox Church in America, applaud the President's initiative in seeking a reasonable compromise between assuring protection of human life at every stage of its development, and exploring the potential therapeutic benefits to be derived from pluripotent stem cells. We are gratified that he has expressed unambiguous opposition to human cloning. We cannot, however, condone the manipulation of embryonic cells in any form for research purposes, including lines developed from destroyed embryos. Rather, we can only express dismay at the fact that the debate over this issue has avoided major considerations regarding the very meaning and value of human life.

President Bush's proposal to use only the existing sixty lines of stem cells[2] because the embryos had already been destroyed (i.e., killed) falters on the precept enunciated by the apostle Paul in Romans 3:8, "We may not do evil so that good may come." The very act of destroying those embryos is evil, and we may not profit from evil even to achieve a good and noble end.

Although the President's Solomonic decision appears to serve pro-life interests, in fact it unwittingly opens the floodgates to ever more utilitarian manipulation of human life. Research on existing stem cell lines should be prohibited for the simple reason that those embryos should never have been created in the first place. The moral line has been crossed, and Mr. Bush's proposed limitations do little to prevent an inevitable descent down an increasingly slippery slope.

Our opposition to ESCR is based on the following considerations, which are political as well as medical and theological.

In the first place, debate on this issue has too often overlooked the fact that among the most vocal proponents of embryo research are pro-abortion activists, supported by much of the media. If the government refuses to fund such research, it would thereby tacitly acknowledge that human life begins at conception. This flies in the face of abortion legislation such as *Roe v. Wade* and would inevitably undermine the view that an embryo is merely a clump of tissue and can therefore be aborted on demand with no moral consequences. The real issue underlying the debate, then, is less the development of potential therapies than the preservation of so-called "abortion rights."[3]

Second, enormous pressures to legalize and federally fund embryonic stem cell research is coming from the biotech and pharmaceutical industries, because of the promise of nearly limitless profits. The "new medicine" based on stem cell therapies is largely driven by the marketplace. As with AIDS medications and other recently developed therapies, market forces will determine who has access to them, and at what cost.

Third, it should be noted that in the recent past (1992) scientists were touting the exceptional benefits of fetal tissue, particularly in the treatment of illnesses such as Parkinson's disease. To date, such therapies have been a disappointment. Some Parkinson's patients, in fact, have suffered irreversible damage due to the introduction of foreign cells into their brains. And no new medicines of significance have been produced using fetal cells. Claims that embryonic stem cells will produce a panacea are likely to be equally exaggerated.

Fourth, the slippery slope of ESCR is dangerous and potentially irreversible. Already an Australian company, in November 2000, received a patent to create chimeras: animals with body tissue and organs produced using human stem cells. And in February 2001, a team of San Francisco researchers announced that they had created a strain of mice, one quarter of whose brains were composed of human cells. In just thirty years the utilitarian slope has taken us from legalized abortion to partial-birth abortion, to physician-assisted suicide and euthanasia, in addition to acceptance of fetal tissue therapy and destruction of embryos to harvest stem cells. Unless moral persuasion can reverse the trend, the slope will lead to a tragic devaluation of human life.

Fifth, ever since the Holocaust the principle has been universally accepted by the scientific community that no experimentation should be undertaken on human subjects without the subject's informed consent. Obviously, such consent cannot be granted by an embryo (nor, by the way, by a two-year old). Neither the mother nor anyone else has "proxy" rights in this regard over the life and well-being of a Child *in utero* or *in vitro*.

Sixth, ESCR relies on cloning to produce multiple copies of the cells under investigation. Cloning in animal experiments has a failure rate on the order of 95%, and mice and other animals produced through cloning have been born with serious genetic defects. The cloning of human embryos for research purposes presents similar dangers, and for this reason alone it should be permanently banned.

Finally, it has been proved recently that adult stem cells, together with those harvested from placentas and umbilical cords, hold as much if not more promise than embryonic stem cells. In May, 2001, the prestigious scientific journal *Cell* published a report showing that adult bone marrow cells have an extraordinary capacity to differentiate into epithelial cells of the liver, lung,

GI tract and skin. The report noted that "This finding may contribute to clinical treatment of genetic disease or tissue repair."[4] In August, 2001, researchers reported finding adult stem cells in mouse brains that were used to produce muscle cells; and a Canadian team isolated "versatile" (pluripotent) cells in mice that produced neural, muscle and fat cells. This means that in the relatively near future it should be possible to harvest stem cells from a patient's skin, multiply them by cloning, and use them for therapeutic purposes, including the growing of new organs.

In conclusion, we firmly reject any and all manipulation of human embryos for research purposes as inherently immoral and a fundamental violation of human life. We call upon the President and the Congress of the United States to restore and maintain a total ban on ESCR. Furthermore, we encourage the scientific community to reject pressures for ESCR exerted by the pro-abortionist lobby, the biotech and pharmaceutical industries, and to devote their energies and resources to discovering, harvesting and utilizing non-embryonic stem cells, including those derived from adults, placentas and umbilical cords.

Above all, we urge our faithful, together with the medical community and political leaders, to return to the spirit of the Hippocratic Oath: primum non nocere, "First of all, do no harm." Embryonic stem cell research results in unmitigated harm. It should be unequivocally rejected in the interests of preserving both the sacredness and the dignity of the human person.

With love in the Lord, the Source of Life,

+THEODOSIUS

Archbishop of Washington

Metropolitan of All America and Canada

And the members of the Holy Synod of Bishops of the Orthodox Church in America:

+KYRILL

Archbishop of Pittsburgh and Western Pennsylvania

+PETER

Archbishop of New York and New Jersey

+DMITRI

Archbishop of Dallas and the South

+HERMAN

Archbishop of Philadelphia and Eastern Pennsylvania

+NATHANIEL

Archbishop of Detroit and the Romanian Episcopate

+JOB
Bishop of Chicago and the Midwest
+TIKHON
Bishop of San Francisco and the West
+SERAPHIM
Bishop of Ottawa and Canada
+NIKOLAI
Bishop of Baltimore
October 17, 2001

Notes

1. J. Breck, *The Sacred Gift of Life* (New York: St. Vladimir's Seminary Press, 1998), chap. 2, "Procreation and the Beginning of Life," pp. 127ff.

2. According to numerous reports, this figure is exaggerated. There may exist throughout the world today only some thirty lines that can prove useful for research purposes. As a result, many scientists are calling for expanding these proposed limitations or for dropping them altogether.

3. This same motivation explains the proliferation of terms to specify discrete stages of life growing in the womb: pre-embryo, embryo, fetus. The reality is that at every stage from conception to birth it is a matter of a human child. Its life is no more "potential" or less human at these stages than is the life of a newborn, a two-year old or an octogenarian.

4. *The National Catholic Bioethics Quarterly*, vol. 1, no. 3 (2001): 443.

Urgent Action Alert: Urge Senators to Support Complete Ban on Human Cloning

UNITED METHODIST CHURCH

T HE ISSUE: Easily available biotechnology has reached the point where some individuals have announced that they are attempting to clone human beings despite aggressive moral, ethical and scientific opposition. Cloning human beings is opposed by over 80% of the US population according to recent polls. In July of this year the House of Representatives approved, by a wide bipartisan margin, and sent to the Senate, the Human Cloning Prohibition Act, HR 2505. As passed in the House, the bill bans all forms of human cloning. The bill has already had its "second reading" and may be brought to the floor for final consideration any time, at the sole discretion of Senate majority leader Tom Daschle (D-SD). The biotechnology industry and special interests anticipating major profits from selling such services and patenting lines of cloned embryos have attempted to confuse the issue with stem cell research, which it has nothing to do with, and to paint the bill as a threat to women's reproductive rights, which over 100 feminists agree it is not.

ACTION NEEDED: Contact both of your Senators and urge them to:

1. Support and vote for the Human Cloning Prohibition Act *as passed in the house* (HR2505 PCS—Similar to S790); and
2. Tell majority leader Daschle that the bill should be brought up for vote immediately.

It is likely that weakening amendments intended to eliminate meaningful penalties and make the ban virtually unenforceable will be offered. Make it clear that you want their support and vote for the clean bill (HR 2505) as passed in the House.

BACKGROUND: Nearly all scientists agree that attempts to clone human beings pose a massive risk of creating large numbers of embryos that will need to be destroyed; producing children who are stillborn, unhealthy, or severely disabled; and subjecting women to unknown risks to their own physical, emotional, and spiritual well-being; and producing children who will almost certainly be prisoners of the expectations of their producers, with little hope for an unfettered possibility to become the unique person God intends.

Creating cloned children begins by creating cloned human embryos, a process which some also propose as a way to create embryos for research or as sources of cells and tissues for possible treatment of other humans. The creation of new human life solely to be exploited and destroyed in this way has been condemned by The United Methodist Church and many others, as displaying a profound disrespect for life. Also, because cloning would take place within the privacy of a doctor-patient relationship, to be effective, a ban on human cloning must stop the cloning process at the beginning. The transfer of embryos to begin a pregnancy is a simple procedure and any government effort to prevent the transfer of an existing embryo or to prevent birth once transfer has occurred would raise substantial moral, legal, and practical issues and will be nearly impossible to implement once cloned embryos are available.

UNITED METHODIST POLICY: As Christians we are called as stewards of creation to till and to keep that which our Creator has made and proclaimed to be good. (Genesis 2) This includes ourselves, as whole, unique, and spiritual persons.

The United Methodist General Conference has said: We call for a ban on all human cloning, including the cloning of human embryos. This includes all projects, privately or governmentally funded, that are intended to advance human cloning. Transcending our concerns with embryo wastage are a number of other unresolved and barely explored concerns with substantial social and theological ramifications: use or abuse of people, exploitation of women, tearing of the fabric of the family, the compromising of human distinctiveness, the lessening of genetic diversity, the direction of research and development being controlled by corporate profit and/or personal gain, and the invasion of privacy. These unresolved concerns generate significant distrust and fear in the general public (*Book of Resolutions 2000*, p. 254).

September 4, 2001

Resolution: On Human Embryonic and Stem Cell Research

SOUTHERN BAPTIST CONVENTION

WHEREAS, Developments in human stem cell research have brought into fresh focus the dignity and status of the human embryo; and

WHEREAS, The National Bioethics Advisory Commission has called for the removal of the ban on public funding of human embryo research; and

WHEREAS, The Bible teaches that human beings are made in the image and likeness of God (Gen. 1:27; 9:6) and protectable human life begins at fertilization; and

WHEREAS, Efforts to rescind the ban on public funding of human embryo research rely on a crass utilitarian ethic which would sacrifice the lives of the few for the benefits of the many; and

WHEREAS, Current law against federal funding of research in which human embryos are harmed and/or destroyed reflects well-established national and international legal and ethical norms against misusing any human being for research purposes; and

WHEREAS, The existing law forbidding public funding of human embryo research is built upon universally held principles governing experiments on human subjects, including principles contained in the Nuremberg Code, the World Medical Association's Declaration of Helsinki, the United Nations Declaration of Human Rights, and other statements; and

WHEREAS, The use of human embryos in research would likely lead to an increase in the number of abortions and create a market for aborted embryos and other fetal tissues; and

WHEREAS, Some forms of human stem cell research require the destruction of human embryos in order to obtain the cells for such research and Southern Baptists are on record for their decades-long opposition to abortion except to save the physical life of the mother and their opposition to destructive human embryo research; and

WHEREAS, Exciting advances in human stem cell research are on the horizon which do not require the destruction of embryos, leading the *British Medical Journal* to state that the use of human embryonic stem cells "may soon be eclipsed by the more readily available and less controversial adult stem cells"; and

WHEREAS, Treatments for Alzheimer's, diabetes, Parkinson's disease, and a host of maladies may soon be within our reach without sacrificing human embryos.

Be it RESOLVED, that we, the messengers to the Southern Baptist Convention, meeting in Atlanta, Georgia, June 15–16, 1999, reaffirm our vigorous opposition to the destruction of innocent human life, including the destruction of human embryos; and

Be it further RESOLVED, that we call upon the United States Congress to maintain the existing ban on the use of tax dollars to support research which requires the destruction of human embryos; and

Be it further RESOLVED, that we call upon those private research centers which perform such experiments to cease and desist from research which destroys human embryos, the most vulnerable members of the human community; and

Be it finally RESOLVED, that we encourage support for the development of alternative treatments which do not require human embryos to be killed.

June 15–16, 1999

Support for Federally Funded Research on Embryonic Stem Cells

UNITED CHURCH OF CHRIST

Background

In the pronouncement on "The Church and Genetic Engineering," the Seventeenth General Synod (1989) noted significant developments in the field of genetics. It spoke of the development of genetics from the foundation of modern genetics by the Austrian monk, Gregor Mendel (1822–1884), to the discovery of the structure of DNA (deoxyribonucleic acid) by James Watson and Francis Crick (1953). Since then research in the field of genetics and genetic engineering has opened new ways to produce products such as insulin, interferon, growth hormones and several other proteins used to treat various diseases. In 1990, the Human Genome Project was initiated by the United States Department of Energy and the National Institutes of Health (NIH) to map and sequence all the genes of human beings by the year 2005. The Genome Project was completed early and last year (2000) the completion of the project was announced with great fan-fare by President Clinton.

A major development in genetics since 1995 has been in the area of human stem cell research. Such research shows great promise for treatment of several diseases which have been nearly untreatable. Stem cells, which can be obtained from embryos, bone marrow, and lymph nodes, are undifferentiated cells, i.e., they have the capability of becoming any type of human cell when properly treated. In 1998 human stem cells were, for the first time, derived from pre-implantation embryos. These cells have been successfully grown for prolonged periods in culture without losing their potential to develop into various human tissues. In addition to advancing basic knowledge in developmental biology, stem cells have practical application, particularly in the fields of transplantation medicine, pharmaceutical research and the development of new drugs. Of particular importance is the promise of new treatments for Juvenile Diabetes, Parkinson's, Alzheimer's, and heart diseases.

Research has shown that embryonic stems cells, i.e., those derived from human embryos, generally those resulting from in vitro fertilization, have greater potential in medical research because they are unlimited in their ability to become various human tissues. While research using embryonic stems cells is opposed by some people, others support such research because of its potential for saving lives and enhancing the quality of life for persons with various diseases. The NIH-established guidelines, known as "National Institutes of Health Guidelines for Research Using Human Pluripotent Stem Cells," were put in place to help ensure that NIH-funded research in this area is conducted in an ethical and legal manner. These guidelines make it clear that NIH funding of research using embryonic stem cells from human embryos can involve only embryos that were created for the purpose of fertility treatment and that were in excess of clinical need. These guidelines were approved by the Clinton administration.

Summary

This resolution calls upon the Twenty-third General Synod of the United Church of Christ to support federally funded embryonic stem cell research. Such research may enable the development of new approaches to diagnosis, prevention, and treatment of some of our most devastating diseases such as Parkinson's, Alzheimer's, Juvenile Diabetes and heart disease.

WHEREAS, Jesus set an example, by his ministry of healing and caring for the sick and disabled, challenging us to follow his example by supporting the healing and caring ministry in our own day, and

WHEREAS, human embryonic stem cells can form virtually any type of human cell and thus have the potential to form tissues for any part of the body, and

WHEREAS, many scientists agree that research on embryonic stem cells is more promising than that of adult stem cells that have only a limited capability to form certain cell types, and

WHEREAS, many scientists believe that embryonic stem cell research could relieve suffering and possibly cure patients with a variety of disorders such as Alzheimer's and Parkinson's diseases, juvenile diabetes, spinal cord injury, Huntington's disease, and muscular dystrophy, and

WHEREAS, there are currently over 25,000 frozen embryos in IVF (in-vitro fertilization) clinics that probably will eventually be discarded, and

WHEREAS, the NIH developed guidelines regulating federally funded research on stem cells, provided they were taken from frozen human embryos derived from in vitro fertilization and which would be discarded after the treatment of infertile couples, and

WHEREAS, in Spring 2001 the present administration canceled the inaugural meeting of a National Institutes of Health (NIH) committee that was to review the applications for federal grants to study human embryonic stem cells; and

WHEREAS, there is bipartisan support for research using human embryos, including many Democratic and Republican legislators, and

WHEREAS, research on embryonic stem cells is already underway in privately funded laboratories where regulations and guidelines do not apply, and

WHEREAS, the support for federally funded research will impose ethical guidelines and oversight, and

WHEREAS, by banning the research, we foreclose the possibility of doing all we can to improve the lot of the living, and in many cases giving them new life,

THEREFORE, BE IT RESOLVED that the Twenty-third General Synod of the United Church of Christ supports federally-funded embryonic stem cell research within ethically sound guidelines (including concern for justice, privacy, access to the benefits of the research for all) and the limitations set forth by the National Institutes of Health, and

BE IT FURTHER RESOLVED that the Twenty-third General Synod requests the General Minister and President of UCC to send a letter to the President of the United States urging approval of federal funding for embryonic stem cell research within NIH guidelines, and

BE IT FURTHER RESOLVED that the Twenty-third General Synod requests Justice and Witness Ministries to advocate for allocation for stem cell research before the appropriate Congressional committees, and

BE IT FURTHER RESOLVED that the Twenty-third General Synod requests Conferences, Association and Local Churches to work diligently in support of the legislation allowing stem cell research, providing appropriate guidelines for such research, and allocating funds to support the research, and

BE IT FURTHER RESOLVED that the Twenty-third General Synod of the United Church of Christ calls upon the Covenanted Ministries to provide leadership and study materials for education, discussion and theological reflection about the ethical issues of developments in the field of stem cell research.

Funding for this action will be made in accordance with the overall mandates of the affected agencies and the funds available.

These resolutions are a part of the minutes of the General Synod. Although the actions have been voted, final approval of the General Synod minutes will occur during the October 2001 meeting of the Executive Council. These minutes will be available in January 2002.

July 2001

Overture 01-50. On Adopting a Resolution Enunciating Ethical Guidelines for Fetal Tissue and Stem Cell Research—From the Presbytery of Baltimore

PRESBYTERIAN CHURCH (USA) RESOLUTION

The Presbytery of Baltimore overtures the 213th General Assembly (2001) to approve the following resolution in accordance the General Assembly Guidelines "Forming Social Policy" paragraph 4:

WHEREAS, the following policy statements of previous General Assemblies of the Presbyterian Church (U.S.A.) provide general guidance that may be considered to apply to fetal tissue and stem cell research:

1. "The Covenant of Life and the Caring Community" (1983), which states, "The 195th General Assembly (1983): . . . Discourages development of human embryos and their use for experimentation except in those cases of clearly demonstrable benefit where no other substitute could accomplish the same end" (Minutes, 1983, Part I, p. 364). The statement goes on to state, "As society looks to the benefits of biotechnology, there must be more serious social and ethical discussion about its application, especially human application. Abuses in eugenics programs in the recent past make the establishment of guidelines for the application of biotechnologies to human beings mandatory. The deepest issues of life and its meaning must not be obscured in the rush to profits and benefits promised by new biotechnologies" (Ibid., p. 365).

2. "Do Justice, Love Mercy, Walk Humbly" (1992), which included the following response to Commissioners' Resolution 89-33 from the 207th General Assembly (1989): "The [General Assembly] concurs

with the intent of the resolution to oppose abortions for the express purpose of selling or providing tissues for research or transplantation, and is opposed to the sale of fetal human tissue obtained in elective abortion. However, we are opposed to, and cannot concur with, calling on Congress to prohibit the use of federal funding for research using fetal tissue" (Minutes, 1992, Part I, p. 373); and

WHEREAS, since these statements were made, both the possible benefits of, and the complicated moral issues involved with, stem cell and fetal tissue research have greatly increased and demand the specific attention of Presbyterians and the larger society; therefore, be it

RESOLVED, That the 213th General Assembly (2001) of the Presbyterian Church (U.S.A.) approves for itself, commends to governing bodies and individual Presbyterians, and presents to the larger society for its consideration the following "Statement on the Ethical and Moral Implications of Stem Cell and Fetal Tissue Research":

Introduction

Contemporary medical research and technologies have presented humankind with complex ethical and moral realities never before envisioned. These realities bear careful review and consideration as new therapies are developed to cure diseases and illnesses. As people of faith we are called to be partners with God in healing and in the alleviation of human pain and suffering.

Human pluripotent stem cells, more commonly known simply as stem cells, are derived through two different methods: one uses early stage embryos in excess of clinical need and donated by women undergoing in vitro fertilization; the other method isolates stem cells from aborted fetuses. Stem cells have the ability to divide for an indefinite period in culture and can develop into most of the specialized cells and tissues of the body, such as muscle cells, nerve cells, liver cells, and blood cells. The use of stem cells has far-reaching possibilities including "cell therapies." Stem cells stimulated to develop into specialized cells could be used to treat diseases such as Parkinson's, Alzheimer's, spinal cord injuries, stroke, burns, heart disease, and diabetes. Using stem cells could reduce the dependence on organ donation and transplantation.

The moral issues raised by stem cell research differ, depending on whether the cells come from aborted fetuses or embryos resulting from in vitro fertilization that are no longer needed for infertility treatment.

Research on Tissue Resulting from Abortion

The ethical acceptability of deriving stem cells from the tissue of aborted fetuses is closely connected to the morality of abortion. Those who oppose using stem cells derived from aborted fetuses argue that abortion for any reason is wrong. Those who so believe also fear that the possibility of donating the fetus for stem cell research will encourage women to have more abortions or justify abortions that otherwise could not be justified. They believe that researchers would be complicit in an immoral act. In addition, they may believe that a woman seeking an abortion should not have the right to give consent to the use of the tissue because she has forfeited her maternal trusteeship by aborting the fetus.

The General Assemblies of the Presbyterian Church (U.S.A.) have consistently supported women's right to choose an abortion based on conscience and religious beliefs. We believe that a woman's right to evaluate her life situation and the impact of her pregnancy on her own health and on her obligations to other family members is an essential element of her personhood and her status as a moral being. We view abortion as not only protected under U.S. law, but as morally justifiable in certain circumstances.

We believe that the use of tissue derived from fetuses is morally and ethically acceptable, provided that the procurement of that tissue is subject to appropriate limitations, and we believe that such limitations should be incorporated into regulatory law. Regulation of donations needs to assure that the decision to have an abortion is separated from the decision to donate fetal tissue. The sale or commercialization of fetal tissue should be legally prohibited.

Research with Stem Cells Derived from Embryos

Research with stem cells obtained from human embryos poses moral difficulties that do not exist in the case of fetal tissues. The life of the fetus has already been terminated when the researcher receives tissue from an aborted fetus, while the life of embryonic tissue resulting from infertility treatment must be terminated. The morality of ending the life of embryos rests on how one views the moral status of the embryos. We believe, as do most authorities that have addressed the issue, that human embryos do have the potential of personhood, and as such they deserve respect. That respect must be shown by requiring that the interests or goals to be accomplished by using human embryos be compelling and unreachable by other means. Indications are that human embryonic stem cell research has the potential to lead to lifesaving breakthroughs in major diseases. Currently, this knowledge cannot be obtained from cells derived from other sources such as adult stem cells and cadaveric fetal tissue. Prohibition of the derivation of stem cells from embryos would elevate the showing of respect to human embryos above that of helping persons whose pain and suffering might be alleviated. Embryos resulting from infertility treatment to be used for such research must be limited to those embryos that do not have a chance of growing into personhood because the woman has decided to discontinue further treatments and they are not available for donation to another woman for personal or medical reasons, or because a donor is not available. Again, the sale or commercialization of embryonic tissue should be legally prohibited.

Conclusion

Therefore, the 213th General Assembly (2001) of the Presbyterian Church (U.S.A.), affirms the use of fetal tissue and embryonic tissue for vital research. Our respect for life includes respect for the embryo and fetus, and we affirm that decisions about embryos and fetuses need to be made with responsibility. Therefore, we believe that the Presbyterian Church (U.S.A.) and other faith groups should educate their members in making these very difficult ethical decisions. With careful regulation, we affirm the use of human stem cell tissue for research that may result in the restoring of health to those suffering from serious illness. We affirm our support for stem cell research, recognizing that this research moves to a new and challenging frontier. We recognize the need for continuing, informed public dialogue and equitable sharing of information of the results of stem cell research. It is only with such public dialogue and information sharing that our diverse society can build a foundation for responsible movement toward this frontier that offers enormous hope and challenge.

Rationale

The present political climate, especially with the change of national administrations, suggests that we may see serious attempts to limit or eliminate fetal tissue and stem cell research.

While the General Assembly has previously opposed the commercialization of fetal tissue and the creation of embryos for research purposes, it has not directly addressed the specific research issues addressed here, though the conclusions stated here can logically be derived from existing policy statements.

The ethical and medical issues are specifically addressed in the resolution.

The proposed statement is based in part on a similar statement adopted by the Board of Directors of the Religious Coalition for Reproduction Choice, August 24, 2000.

ACSWP ADVICE AND COUNSEL ON OVERTURE 01-50

Advice and Counsel on Overture 01-50—From the Advisory Committee on Social Witness Policy (ACSWP).

Overture 01-50 proposes approving a resolution that enunciates ethical guidelines for fetal tissue and stem cell research, building on previous General Assembly policies.

The Advisory Committee on Social Witness Policy advises that the Overture 01-50 is consistent with previous General Assembly policies.

Rationale: Overture 01-50 is proposed to General Assembly in the form of a resolution. A resolution "applies existing policy statements to new circumstances" ("Why and How the Church Makes a Social Policy Witness," *Minutes,* 1993, Part I, p. 768). The development of a resolution requires that there is adequate policy so that policy can be applied to current societal realities.

This resolution accurately builds on policies of past General Assemblies. The second "Whereas" refers to: "Abortion is not morally acceptable for gender selection only or solely to obtain fetal parts for transplantation" (*Minutes,* 1992, Part I, p. 368). An additional statement, made in response to Commissioners' Resolution 89-33 *(Minutes,* 1992, Part I, p. 373), is accurately quoted in Overture 01-50.

The 195th General Assembly (1983) stated that it "Discourages development of human embryos and their use for experimentation except in those cases of clearly demonstrable benefit where no other substitute could accomplish the same end" (*Minutes,* 1983, Part I, p. 361). The overture includes another direct quote from the 195th General Assembly (1983) that declares the need for establishing guidelines for this work (*Minutes,* 1983, Part I, p. 365). Overture 01-50 proposes one step in developing those guidelines.

Stem cell research continues to develop very rapidly. A lot of research is underway using cells from umbilical cords and adult cell types. Highly promising and significant progress is reported weekly. However, at this time and in the near future, most of the stem cells will continue to be derived from early stage embryos and aborted fetuses. Therefore, scientists believe that all avenues of research should remain open.

[Available at http://www.pcusa.org/ga213/business/OVT0150.htm]
June 2001

A Theologian's Brief on the Place of the Human Embryo within the Christian Tradition, and the Theological Principles for Evaluating Its Moral Status

Submitted to the House of Lords Select Committee on Stem Cell Research by an ad hoc group of Christian theologians from the Anglican, Catholic, Orthodox and Reformed traditions.

Basis of this Submission

1. In a multi-cultural and multi-religious society, it is appropriate to take account not only of secular arguments concerning the place of the human embryo but also of arguments expressed in the religious language of some sections of the community. It is particularly important to understand the *Christian* tradition in this regard because of the place Christianity has had in shaping the moral understanding of many citizens in this country, and because this tradition has already been invoked in the context of public debate.[1]

2. The Human Fertilisation and Embryology (Research Purposes) Regulations 2001 greatly expand the purposes for which research using human embryos can take place, and thus, if implemented, will inevitably lead to a massive increase in the use and destruction of embryos. The Select Committee has expressed its wish not "to review the underlying basis of the 1990 Act";[2] however, the ethical and legal issues surrounding "the Regulations as they now stand" *cannot* adequately be addressed without considering the moral status of the human embryo. Similarly, the "regulatory framework established by the 1990 Act" *cannot* operate effectively if it is flawed in principle.

3. Adding more purposes for which human embryos can be created for destructive use builds upon a mistake that has already been made in the existing legislation. By far the most important ethical issue involved in the Regulations "as they now stand" relates to the ethical significance of embryonic human individuals whether produced by cloning or by the ordinary process of fertilization. The spectacle of thousands of stock-piled frozen human embryos being destroyed at the behest of this legislation bore witness that, even in the area of fertility treatment, too little consideration had been given to regulating the initial production of human embryos, as opposed to their subsequent disposal. The Regulations 2001 make the situation even worse in this regard.

The Christian Tradition

4. Some scholars, considering the prospective benefits to be derived from experimenting on human embryos, have alleged that the Christian tradition had already set a precedent for treating the early human embryo with "graded status and protection."[3] In support of this it has been noted that there were seventh century books of penance ("Penitentials") which graded the level of penance for abortion according to whether the foetus was "formed" or "unformed." The same distinction was invoked in Roman Catholic canon law which, from 1591 to 1869, imposed excommunication only for the abortion of a "formed" foetus. Furthermore, St. Thomas Aquinas, one of the most authoritative theologians of the Middle Ages, explicitly held that the human embryo did not possess a spiritual soul and was not a human being (*homo*) until forty days in the case of males or ninety in the case of females.[4] Texts from the Fathers of the Church could easily be found to support a similar conclusion.

5. Nevertheless, the contention that for most of Christian history (until 1869) the human embryo has been considered to possess only a relative value—such as might be outweighed by considerations of the general good—relies on a misreading of the tradition. Even in the Middle Ages, when most Western Christians held that the early embryo was not yet fully human, it was held that the human embryo should never be attacked deliberately, however extreme the circumstances. To gain the proper historical perspective it is necessary to supply a wider context by incorporating other elements of that tradition.

6. The earliest Christian writings on the issue declared simply, "you shall not murder a child by abortion":[5] the embryo was held to be inviolable at

every stage of its existence.[6] The first Christian writings to consider the question of when human life began asserted that the spiritual soul was present from conception.[7] As one account puts it: "The Early Church adopted a critical attitude to the widespread practice of abortion and infanticide. It did so on the basis of a belief in the sanctity of human life; a belief which was in turn an expression of its faith in the goodness of creation and of God's particular care for humankind."[8]

7. The earliest Church legislation also contains no reference to the distinction of formed and unformed,[9] and St. Basil the Great, who did consider it, saw it as a sophistical exercise in splitting hairs: "We do not consider the fine distinction between formed and unformed."[10]

8. In the fourth and fifth centuries some theologians argued that human life began at conception,[11] some held that the spiritual soul was "infused" at forty days or so[12] (following Aristotle)[13] and some held that the timing of the infusion of the soul was a mystery known to God alone.[14] However, whatever their views about the precise moment when human life began, all Christians held that abortion was gravely wrong,[15] an offense against God the Creator and either the killing of a child, or something very like the killing of a child. If it was not regarded as homicide in the strict sense, "it was looked upon as anticipated homicide, or interpretive homicide, or homicide in intent, because it involved the destruction of a future man. It was always closely related to homicide."[16]

9. In the Anglo Saxon and Celtic "Penitentials" (from the seventh century) and in the canon law of the Latin Church (from the eleventh century) abortion of a formed foetus sometimes carried heavier penalties than did abortion of an unformed foetus. Yet canon law has an eye not just on objective harm done but also on subjective culpability and on enforceability. The decision of Gregory XIV in 1591 to limit the penalty of excommunication to the abortion of a formed foetus was expressly due to problems enforcing earlier legislation.[17] Abortion of an unformed foetus was sometimes regarded as, technically, a different sin—and sometimes (though not universally) as a lesser sin—than abortion of a formed foetus, but it continued to be regarded as a grave sin closely akin to homicide.

10. From the twelfth century until the seventeenth century, convinced by the anatomy of Galen and the philosophy of Aristotle, most Christians in the West came to believe that the spiritual soul was infused forty days or so after conception. Nevertheless, during this whole period, there was no suggestion that the unformed foetus was expendable. The unformed foetus continued to be regarded as sacrosanct. It was *never* seen as legitimate to harm the

embryo directly, only incidentally, and only then in the course of trying to save the mother's life.[18]

11. The first theologian to suggest explicitly that the embryo had a graded moral status, that is, a relative value that could be outweighed by other values, was Thomas Sanchez in the late sixteenth century.[19] He and other "laxists" proposed that a woman could legitimately abort an unformed foetus to avoid public shame of a kind which might endanger her life. This suggestion constituted a radical departure from the thinking of previous moralists such as St. Raymond of Penafort or St. Antoninus of Florence and provoked the criticism of Sanchez's contemporaries, the scandal of the faithful and, in 1679, the condemnation of Pope Innocent XI.[20]

12. Between this discredited school of the seventeenth century and the re-emergence of similar views in the late twentieth century, there is no significant or continuous strand of Christian tradition—either in the Catholic or the Reformed churches. The most balanced and representative Catholic moralist of the eighteenth century, St. Alphonsus Liguori, allowed no exception to the prohibition on "direct" (intentional) abortion and allowed "indirect" (unintentional) abortion only in the context of attempting to save the mother's life. In a statement reminiscent of St. Basil he declared that the distinction of formed and unformed made no practical difference.[21] He is the last great moralist to consider the inviolability of the "unformed" foetus as such, because, during his time, the prevailing medical opinion moved away from the distinction between formed and unformed. In his later writing (on baptism) St. Alphonsus also became sympathetic to the view that the spiritual soul was infused at conception.[22]

13. From the seventeenth century the classical biology of Galen and Aristotle had begun to be displaced by a variety of other theories. One, in particular, gave a more equal role to the female and male elements in generation, and therefore increased the significance of "fertilization," that is, the moment of the union of male and female gametes.[23] This theory was finally confirmed in 1827 with the first observation of a mammalian ovum under the microscope, a scientific development which informed the decision of Pius IX in 1869 to abolish the distinction in legal penalties between early and late abortions. By the mid-nineteenth century the prevailing opinion, among both Reformed and Roman Catholic Christians, was that, most probably, the spiritual soul was infused at conception.[24]

14. In asserting that "life must be protected with the utmost care from conception"[25] and rejecting "the killing of a life already conceived,"[26] twen-

tieth century Christians were in continuity with the belief of the Early Church that all human life is sacred from conception. This had remained a *constant* feature of Christian tradition despite a variety of beliefs about the origin of the soul and a similar variety in what legal penalties were thought appropriate for early or late abortion.[27]

15. In the tradition, the only precedents for attributing a "graded status and protection" to the embryo can be found in the speculations of some of the Roman Catholic laxists of the seventeenth century and the re-emergence of similar and even more radical views among some Protestant and Roman Catholic writers in the late twentieth century.[28] The great weight of the tradition, East and West, Orthodox, Catholic and Reformed, from the apostolic age until the twentieth century, is firmly against any sacrifice or destructive use of the early human embryo save, perhaps, "at the dictate of strict and undeniable medical necessity";[29] that is, in the context of seeking to save the mother's life.

Some Theological Principles

16. For a Christian, the question of the status of the human embryo is directly related to the mystery of creation. In the context of the creation of things "seen and unseen"[30] the human being appears as the *microcosm*, reflecting in the unity of a single creature both spiritual and corporeal realities.[31] The beginning of each human being is therefore a reflection of the coming to be of the world as a whole. It reveals the creative act of God bringing about the reality of *this* person (of me), in an analogous way to the creation of the entire cosmos. There is a mystery involved in the existence of each person.

17. Often in the Scriptures the forming of the child in the womb is described in ways that echo the formation of Adam from the dust of the earth.[32] This is why Psalm 139 describes the child in the womb as being formed "in the depths of the earth."[33] The formation of the human embryo is archetypal of the mysterious works of God.[34] A passage that is significant for uncovering the connections between Genesis and embryogenesis is found in the deutero-canonical book of Maccabees, in a mother's speech to her son:

I do not know how you came into being in my womb. It was not I who gave you life and breath, nor I who set in order the elements within each of you. Therefore the Creator of the world, who shaped the beginning of man and devised the origin of all things, will in his mercy give life and breath back to you again.[35]

18. The book of Genesis marks out human beings from other creatures. Only human beings—male and female—are described as being made in "the image and likeness of God"; only they are given dominion over creation; only Adam is portrayed as receiving life from God's breath and as naming the animals.[36] However, at the same time, it is clear that human beings are earthly creatures, made on the same day as other land animals, made from the dust of the earth, not descending out of heaven. Because they are earthly, human beings are mortal: "Dust you are and to dust you will return."[37] There is no sign in these stories of the dualism of body and soul that is found in Pythagoras or in the ancient mystery religions. The soul is not a splinter of God that is trapped in a body. The soul is the natural life of the body, given by the life-giving God.

19. It was because of the Jewish conviction of the unity of the human being that, when hope was kindled within Israel for a life beyond the grave, it was expressed as a hope for the resurrection of the *body*.[38] The disembodied life of the shades in the gloomy underworld of Sheol[39] was not an image of hope but an image of death. The resurrection of the body was presented as the triumph of the Lord over death, the vindication of those who had been faithful to the Lord, even unto death,[40] and for Christians was given new meaning and foundation in the resurrection of Jesus.[41] The story of the empty tomb and the description of the resurrection appearances emphasized the bodily reality of the life of the resurrection. Jesus walked with the disciples and ate with them and invited them to touch his hands and his feet. "Handle me and see that I am no bodiless phantom."[42]

20. The Fathers of the Church attempted to do justice to the scriptural truths of the bodily resurrection and of the mysterious parallel between the origin of each human individual and the origin of the entire cosmos. From different competing beliefs, the doctrine which prevailed was that the spiritual *soul*—what makes each individual human person unique, and gives each one the ability to know and to love—is neither generated by the parents nor does it pre-exist the body, but it is created directly by God with the coming to be of each human being.[43] Throughout the history of the Church, Christians have used the language of "body and soul" to understand the human being, but in such a way as not to deny the unity of God's creation. In the fourteenth century, in an attempt to defend this human unity, the Ecumenical Council of Vienne defined the doctrine that the soul was "the form of

the body" (*forma corporis*),[44] by which it meant: what gives life to the body. Christians held, and continue to hold, that the spiritual soul is present from the moment there is a living human body[45] until the time that body dies.

21. The Scriptures also emphasize how God's provident care for each person is present before he or she is ever aware of it. The Lord called his prophets by name before they were born: "The Lord called me from the womb, from the body of my mother he named my name."[46] "Before I formed you in the womb I knew you, and before you were born I consecrated you."[47] It is possible to understand these passages as referring not only to the prophets, but to each one of God's children. The Lord calls each one from the womb, forms each one, gives each one into the care of his or her mother, and will not abandon his creature in times of trial.[48]

> For it was you who created my being, knit me together in my mother's womb.
> I thank you for the wonder of my being, for the wonders of all your creation.
> Already you knew my soul my body held no secret from you when I was being fashioned in secret and moulded in the depths of the earth.[49]

22. Such passages do not establish *when* human life begins, but they establish God's involvement and care from the very *beginning*, a concern that is not diminished by our lack of awareness of him.

23. "In reality it is only in the mystery of the Word made flesh that the mystery of the human being truly becomes clear."[50] To illuminate the mystery of the origin of human persons it seems reasonable to turn to the mystery of the Incarnation. In order to do justice to the infancy narratives, especially that of the Gospel of Luke, one must believe that, from the moment of the Annunciation to Mary of Jesus's birth, Mary conceived by the Holy Spirit and carried the Saviour in her womb. This is emphasized by the story of the Visitation—where one pregnant mother greets another, and the unborn John bears witness to the unborn Jesus.

24. The Incarnation was revealed to the world at the Nativity when Jesus was born, but the Incarnation *began* at the Annunciation, when the Word took flesh and came to dwell within the womb of the Virgin. This understanding of the text of Scripture is confirmed by the witness of the Fathers of the Church,[51] by the development of the feast of the Annunciation and, not least, by the solemn declaration of the Fourth Ecumenical Council, the Council of Chalcedon (451 CE):

We profess the holy Virgin to be Mother of God, for God the Word became flesh and was made man and from the moment of conception (ex auteis teis sulleipseoes/*ex ipso conceptu*) united himself to the temple he had taken from her.[52]

25. In the Eastern Church, St. Maximus the Confessor turned to the Annunciation[53] to illuminate the intractable problem of when human life begins. Jesus is said to have been like to us in all things but sin[54] and Christians believe that Jesus was a human being from the moment of conception: therefore, it seems, every human being must come into existence at the moment of conception.

26. In the West, Christians were more strongly influenced by the biology of Galen and the philosophy of Aristotle and held that the spiritual soul was only infused at the moment when the body was perfectly formed, forty days after conception. The great medieval Christian thinkers all held that the conception of Jesus was an exception, and that he was *unlike* us in the womb.[55] This was an unhappy conclusion, forced upon theologians by an erroneous biology. Is it really sustainable to argue that Jesus was unlike us in his humanity? A more adequate vision was supplied by the seventeenth century Anglican theologian Lancelot Andrewes, in a sermon on the Nativity:

For our conception being the root as it were, the very groundsill of our nature; that he might go to the root and repair our nature from the very foundation, thither he went.[56]

27. The words of this sermon bring our attention, not only to the work of the Redeemer from the beginning of his life, but also to our need for redemption from the beginning of our lives. It was this need that David recognized in himself according to the psalm, "Behold, I was brought forth in iniquity, and in sin did my mother conceive me,"[57] where these words refer not to his mother's sinfulness, but to the complete extent of his own sinfulness. This psalm and the Eden story were given a deeper sense by Christians in light of the redemption accomplished by Jesus. As Jesus had achieved a total transformation, so all human beings were in need of a total transformation: total in the sense of including their very origins. In his letter to the Romans, St. Paul drew out the parallel between Adam and Christ and so asserted the involvement of all human beings in Adam's sin.[58]

28. This association of sin and conception is also shown within the Roman Catholic tradition in the development of the doctrine of Mary's complete redemption from sin. The doctrine of the Immaculate Conception appears to imply that Mary was receptive to grace from the moment of her conception in her mother's womb. This Roman Catholic argument is simply an expression of a more widely accepted argument from the Christian doctrine of original sin. Both arguments express the general truth that each and every human being needs the help of God from the very first—which is constantly and, it seems, inevitably expressed as "from the first moment of his or her conception."

29. The Christian churches teach not that the early embryo is certainly a person, but that the embryo should always be treated *as if* it were a person.[59] This is not only a case of giving the embryo the benefit of the doubt—refraining from what might be the killing of an innocent person. It is also that the ambiguity in the appearance of the embryo has never been thought of as taking the embryo out of the realm of the human, the God-made and the holy. When Pope John Paul II asks, "how can a human individual not be a human person?"[60] he is not denying the mysteriousness of the implied answer. Christians recognize the embryo to be sacred precisely because it is inseparable from the mystery of the creation of the human person by God.[61] What is clear, at the very least, is that the embryo is "a living thing—under the care of God."[62]

30. The following, then, are five principal considerations which should inform any Christian evaluation of the moral status of the human embryo:

I.   Though penalties have varied, the Christian tradition has always extended the principle of the sacredness of human life to the very beginning of each human being, and never allowed the deliberate destruction of the fruit of conception.

II. The origin of each human being is not only a work of nature but is a special work of God in which God is involved from the very beginning.

III. The Christian doctrine of the soul is not dualistic but requires one to believe that, where there is a living human individual, there is a spiritual soul.

IV. Each human being is called and consecrated by God in the womb from the first moment of his or her existence, before he or she becomes aware of it. Traditionally, Christians have expressed the human need for redemption as extending from the moment of conception.

V.   Jesus, who reveals to Christians what it is to be human, was a human individual from the moment of his conception, celebrated on the feast of the Annunciation, nine months before the feast of Christmas.

31. Jesus reveals the humanity especially of the needy and those who have been overlooked. Concern over the fate of embryos destined for research is inspired, not only by the narratives of the Annunciation, the Visitation and the Nativity, but also by the parable of the good Samaritan and the parable of the sheep and the goats: "Just as you did it to one of the least of these little ones you did it to me."[63] The aim of an ethically serious amendment to the 1990 Act should be to regulate the procedures in fertility treatment and non-destructive medical research on human embryos such that these human individuals are adequately protected.

Prepared by **Rev. David Jones** MA MA MSt, Director of the Linacre Centre for Healthcare Ethics, London.

On behalf of an ad hoc group of Christian theologians from the Anglican, Catholic, Orthodox and Reformed traditions and endorsed by:

+ **Cardinal Cahal B. Daly**, BA MA DD, Peritus at Vatican II, Archbishop Emeritus of Armagh, Primate Emeritus of All Ireland.

+ **Rt. Rev. Kallistos Ware**, MA DPhil, Bishop of Diokleia in the Orthodox Archdiocese of Thyateira and Great Britain, Lecturer in Eastern Orthodox Studies, Oxford University.

+ **Most Rev. Rowan Williams**, MA DPhil DD, FBA, Bishop of Monmouth, Archbishop of Wales.

Rev. Prof. Benedict M. Ashley OP, MA STL PhD PhD STM, Adjunct Professor, Center for Healthcare Ethics, St. Louis University, St. Louis, Missouri.

Dr. Margaret Atkins, MA MA PhD, Lecturer in Theology, Trinity and All Saints College, Leeds.

Rev. Prof Michael Banner, BA DPhil, Professor of Moral and Social Theology, King's College, London.

Rev. Prof. Nigel M. de S. Cameron, MA BD PhD, Professor of Theology and Culture, Trinity International University, Illinois.

Prof. Celia Deane-Drummond, BA MA PhD PhD, Professor in Theology and the Biological Sciences, Chester College, University of Liverpool.

Prof. Michael J. Gorman, BA MDiv PhD, Dean, The Ecumenical Institute of Theology, Professor of New Testament and Early Church History, St. Mary's University and Seminary, Baltimore, Maryland.

Prof. Vigen Guroian, BA PhD, Professor of Theology and Ethics, Loyola College, Baltimore, Maryland, Visiting Lecturer, St. Nersess Armenian Seminary.

Prof. Andrew Louth, MA MA MTh DD, Professor of Patristic and Byzantine Studies, University of Durham.

Prof. William E May, BA MA PhD, Professor of Moral Theology, John Paul II Institute for Marriage and Family, Washington.

Rev. Herbert McCabe OP, STL BA STM, Lecturer in Theology, Blackfriars Hall, Oxford.

Prof. Gilbert Meilaender, BA MDiv PhD, Professor of Christian Ethics, Valparaiso, Indiana.

Prof. John Milbank, BA MA PhD DD, Professor of Philosophical Theology, University of Virginia.

Dr. C. Ben Mitchell, BS MDiv PhD, Senior Fellow, The Center for Bioethics & Human Dignity, Bannockburn, Illinois.

Rev. Dr. Aidan Nichols OP, STL MA DipTheol PhD, Affiliated lecturer, Divinity Faculty, Cambridge University, Lecturer in Theology, Blackfriars Hall, Oxford.

Rev. Prof. Oliver O'Donovan, MA DPhil, Canon of Christi Church, Regius Professor of Moral and Pastoral Theology, Oxford University.

Rev. Terence Phipps MA AM STL, Lecturer in Moral Theology, Allen Hall, London.

Prof. John Rist, MA, FRSC, Professor Emeritus, University of Toronto, Visiting Professor, Institutum Patristicum Augustinianum, Rome.

Prof. John Saward, BA MLitt, Professor of Dogmatic Theology, International Theological Institute, Gaming Austria, Aquinas Fellow, Plater College, Oxford.

Dr. Robert Song, MA DPhil, Lecturer in Theology, University of Durham.

Rev. Dr. Thomas G Weinandy OFMCap, BA MA MA PhD, Warden, Tutorial Fellow in Theology, Greyfriars, Oxford.

Submitted to the House of Lords, 1st June 2001.

Notes

1. Hansard Vol. 62 1, No.16, col. 35.37.
2. In its "Call for Evidence."
3. Cf. G. R. Dunstan "The Human Embryo in the Western Moral Tradition" in G. R.

Dunstan and M. J. Sellers *The Status of the Human Embryo* London: King Edward's Hospital Fund, 1988, p. 55.

4. *Commentary on the Sentences* book IV, d. 31 exp. text.

5. *Didache* 2.2; *Epistle of Barnabas* 19.5.

6. See also *Apocalypse of Peter* 2.26; St. Clement of Alexandria *Teacher* II.10.96; *Athenagoras Legatio* 35; Municius Felix Octavius 30.2; Tertullian *Apology* 9.4–8; Hippolytus *Refutation of All Heresies* 9.7.

7. St. Clement *Prophetic Eclogues* 41, 48–49, cf. M. J. Gorman *Abortion and the Early Church: Christian, Jewish & Pagan Attitudes in the Greco-Roman World* Downers Grove Ill.: InterVarsity Press, 1982, p. 52; Tertullian *On the Soul* 27. "Now we allow that life begins with conception, because we contend that the soul also begins from conception; life taking its commencement at the same moment and place that the soul does."

8. "Some Current Ethical Issues Concerning the Treatment of the Pre-Implantation Human Embryo," a briefing paper prepared by the General Synod Board for Social Responsibility; cf. G. Bonner, "Abortion and Early Christian Thought" in J. H. Channer ed. *Abortion and the Sanctity of Human Life,* Exeter: The Paternoster Press, 1985; M. J. Gorman "Abortion and the Early Church" at http://www.incommunion.org/gorman.htm; L. Crutchfield "The Early Church Fathers and Abortion" at http://www.all.org/issues/ab99x.htm.

9. Elvira (305 CE) canons 53, 65; Ancyra (314 CE) 21; Lerida (524 CE) 2; Braga (527 CE) 77; Trullo (692 CE) 91; Mainz (847 CE) 21; cf. S. Troianos "The Embryo in Byzantine Canon Law" http://business.hol.gr/~bio/allfile/HTML/PUBS/VOL3/ha-trx.htm.

10. Basil Epistle 118.2.

11. St. Gregory of Nyssa *On the Making of Man* 29; cf. St. Maximus the Confessor II *Ambigua* 42.

12. Lactantius *De Opificio Dei* 12; Ambrosiaster QQ *Veteris et Novi Testamenti* 23.

13. *On the History of Animals* VII.3, 4:583.

14. St. Jerome *On Ecclesiastes* 2.5; *Apologia adversus Rufinum* 2.8; St. Augustine *Enchiridion* 85, *On Exodus* 2.80; though each of these sometimes state that the foetus is not a man (homo) until he is fully formed.

15. St. Augustine *On Marriage and Concupiscence* 1.15; St. Ambrose *Hexameron* 5.18; St. Jerome *Epistle* 22, 13; St. John Chrysostom *Homily 24 on the Epistle to the Romans*; Caesarius of Arles *Sermons* 9, 91.

16. J. Connery, *Abortion: The Development of the Roman Catholic Perspective,* Chicago: Loyola University Press, 1977, p. 306, cf. G. Grisez, *Abortion: the Myths the Realities and the Arguments,* New York: Corpus Books, 1970; J. T. Noonan "An Almost Absolute Value in History" in J. T. Noonan ed. *The Morality of Abortion: Legal and Historical Perspectives* Cambridge Mass.: Harvard University Press, 1970.

17. Bull of 1591, *Sedes Apostolica* cf. Connery p. 148; Grisez pp. 167–168; Noonan p. 33.

18. Connery pp. 114–134; Grisez pp. 166–168; Noonan pp. 26–27.

19. Connery pp. 134–141; Grisez pp. 168–169; Noonan pp. 27–31.

20. Denzinger-Schoenmetzer *Enchiridion Symbolorum* Rome: Herder, 1965, 2134–2135 cf. Connery p. 189; Grisez p. 174; Noonan p. 34.

21. *Theologia Moralis* III, 4.1, n. 394.

22. *Theologia Moralis* VI, 1.1, dubia 4, n. 124 cf. Connery p. 210; Grisez p. 176; Noonan p. 31.

23. The theory developed by Fienus (1567–1631), Zacchia (1584–1659) and Cangiamila (1701–1763) cf. Connery ch. 10–11; Grisez pp. 170–172; Noonan pp. 34–40.

24. This has also become the prevailing opinion among followers of St. Thomas Aquinas, cf. B. Ashley "A Critique of the Theory of Delayed Hominization" in McCarthy D., Moraczewski, A., *Evaluation of Fetal Experimentation: An Interdisciplinary Study* St. Louis: Pope John Center, 1976; B. Ashley and A. Moraczewski "Cloning, Aquinas, and the Embryonic Person" *The National Catholic Bioethics Quarterly* 1 (2000), 189–201; S. Heaney, "Aquinas and the Presence of the Human Rational Soul in the Early Embryo" *The Thomist* 56, (1992) 1; M. Johnston "Delayed Hominization" *Theological Studies* 56 (1995); R. Joyce "The Human Zygote Is a Person" *The New Scholasticism* 51 (1975).

25. Second Vatican Council *Gaudium et Spes* 51.

26. Lambeth Conference 1958 report "The Family in Contemporary Society" in *What the Bishops Have Said about Marriage* London: SPCK, 1968, p. 17.

27. "The Church has always held in regard to the morality of abortion that it is a serious sin to destroy a fetus at any stage of development. However, as a *juridical norm* in the determination of penalties against abortion, the Church at various times did accept the distinction between a *formed* and a *non-formed,* an *animated* and a *nonanimated* fetus." R. J. Huser *The Crime of Abortion in Canon Law* Washington D.C.: Catholic Univ. Press, 1942, preliminary note.

28. An ill-tempered but perceptive critique of some recent attempts to reread the Christian tradition on abortion as "relatively tolerant" to abortion of an unformed foetus is D. DeMarco "The Roman Catholic Church and Abortion: An Historical Perspective" in *Homiletic & Pastoral Review* July 1984, 59–66 and August–September, 68–76; cf. http://www.petersnet.net/research/retrieve.cfm?RecNum=3362.

29. Lambeth Conference 1958 report "The Family in Contemporary Society" in *What the Bishops Have Said about Marriage* London: SPCK, 1968, p. 17.

30. Creed of Nicaea, N. Tanner *Decrees of the Ecumenical Councils* London: Sheed & Ward, 1990, I. p. 5.

31. Gregory of Nyssa *On the Making of Man;* John Damascene *Exposition of the Orthodox Faith* II.12; Creed of Lateran IV, Tanner p. 230.

32. Job 10.8–12, Ecclesiastes 11.5, Ezekiel 37.7–10, (cf. Wisdom 7.1, 15.10–11).

33. Psalm 139.15.

34. Psalm 139.15, Ecclesiastes 11.5.

35. II Maccabees 7.22–23.

36. Genesis 1.26–28; 2.7; 2.19–20.

37. Genesis 3.19.

38. Daniel 12.2–3; cf. Ezekiel 37.1–14; John 11.24.

39. Job 10.21–22; Psalms 6.5, 88.10, 115.17; Ecclesiastes 9.3–6 cf. Homer *Odyssey* XI. 485–491.

40. Isaiah 26.19; Hosea 13.14; (cf. II Maccabees 7.9–14).

41. John 11.1–44.

42. Ignatius of Antioch *Smyrneans* 3 cf. Luke 24:13–51; John 20.19–29.

43. John Damascene, Peter Lombard, St. Thomas Aquinas *Summa Theologiae* Ia Q. 118 art. 2–3; Pius XII *Humani Generis.*

44. Council of Vienne, *On the Catholic Faith,* Tanner p. 361.

45. The debate about the timing of the "infusion of the soul" was a debate about when the living human body came into existence.

46. Isaiah 49.1.

47. Jeremiah 1.5.

48. Psalm 22.10–11; Psalm 71.6; Job 10.8–12.

49. Psalm 139.

50. Second Vatican Council, *Gaudium et Spes* 22.

51. J. Saward *The Redeemer in the Womb* San Francisco: Ignatius, 1993, ch. 3.

52. Epistle of St. Cyril to John of Antioch, Tanner p. 70.

53. *II Ambigua* 42.

54. Hebrews 4.15.

55. Cf. Thomas Aquinas *Summa Theologiae* IIIa Q.6 art. 4.

56. Sermon IX on the Nativity in J. Saward, p. 100.

57. Psalm 51.5.

58. Romans 5.12–21.

59. For example, "The human being is to be respected and treated as a person from the moment of conception" Pope John Paul II *Evangelium Vitae* 60, emphasis added.

60. Ibid.

61. Cf. O. O'Donovan *Begotten or Made?* Oxford: Clarendon Press, 1984, ch. 4.

62. Athenagoras *Legatio* 35.

63. Matthew 25.40.

Cloning Research, Jewish Tradition and Public Policy: A Joint Statement by the Union of Orthodox Jewish Congregations of America and the Rabbinical Council of America

Society today stands on the threshold of a new era in biomedical research. The wisdom granted to humans by our Creator has led to our greater understanding and knowledge of the building blocks of human life itself. Scientists revealed the existence and role of DNA and cellular science many years ago. Currently, scientists are not only able to describe the nature of cellular life, but manipulate it as well. We are now faced with the possibility of mastering the art of this manipulation to the point of being able to clone in research laboratories the cells that, in other circumstances, lead to fully developed human beings.

A debate has emerged in American society at large and among our elected leaders as to whether public policy should permit, encourage, restrict or ban the further conduct of this biomedical research. The issue is one with complex moral dimensions. On the one hand scientific research indicates that there is great life-saving potential in the results that can come from cloning research. On the other hand, we must be vigilant against any erosion of the value that society accords to human life.

Our Torah tradition places great value upon human life; we are taught in the opening chapters of Genesis that each human was created in God's image. After creating man and woman, God empowered them to enter a partnership with Him in the stewardship of the world. The Torah commands us to treat and cure the ill and to defeat disease wherever possible; to do this is to be the Creator's partner in safeguarding the created. The traditional Jewish perspective thus emphasizes that maximizing the potential to save and heal human lives is an integral part of valuing human life. Moreover, our tradition states that an embryo *in vitro* does not enjoy the full status of human-hood and its attendant protections. Thus, if cloning technology research advances our ability to heal humans with greater success, it ought to be pursued since it does not require or encourage the destruction of life in the process.

However, cloning research must not be pursued indiscriminately. We must be careful to distinguish between cloning for therapeutic purposes—which ought to be pursued—and cloning for reproductive purposes—which we oppose. Thus, this research must be conducted under strict guidelines and with strict limitations to ensure that the research is indeed serving therapeutic purposes.

Consistent with this policy, we advocate that a fully funded and empowered oversight body comprised of scientists and ethicists be created to monitor this research. Relevant Executive-branch agencies and congressional committees should conduct periodic reviews as well. The oversight process should pay special attention to ensuring that the embryos used in this research are not brought to a point which constitutes human-hood.

We believe that the policy stated herein articulates the perspective of the Torah tradition and the community we represent and achieves the correct balance between pursuing new methods for saving human lives and maintaining the fundamental respect and sanctity of human life.

Human Cloning and Human Dignity: An Ethical Inquiry

THE PRESIDENT'S COUNCIL ON BIOETHICS
WASHINGTON, D.C.

Executive Summary

For the past five years, the prospect of human cloning has been the subject of considerable public attention and sharp moral debate, both in the United States and around the world. Since the announcement in February 1997 of the first successful cloning of a mammal (Dolly the sheep), several other species of mammals have been cloned. Although a cloned human child has yet to be born, and although the animal experiments have had low rates of success, the production of functioning mammalian cloned offspring suggests that the eventual cloning of humans must be considered a serious possibility.

In November 2001, American researchers claimed to have produced the first cloned human embryos, though they reportedly reached only a six-cell stage before they stopped dividing and died. In addition, several fertility specialists, both here and abroad, have announced their intention to clone human beings. The United States Congress has twice taken up the matter, in 1998 and again in 2001–2002, with the House of Representatives in July 2001 passing a strict ban on all human cloning, beginning with the production of cloned human embryos. As of this writing, several cloning-related bills are under consideration in the Senate. Many other nations have banned human cloning, and the United Nations is considering an international convention on the subject. Finally, two major national reports have been issued on human reproductive cloning, one by the National Bioethics Advisory Commission (NBAC) in 1997, the other by the National Academy of Sciences (NAS) in

January 2002. Both the NBAC and the NAS called for further consideration of the ethical and social questions raised by cloning.

The debate over human cloning became further complicated in 1998
when researchers were able, for the first time, to isolate human embryonic
stem cells. Many scientists believe that these versatile cells, capable of becoming any type of cell in the body, hold great promise for understanding
and treating many chronic diseases and conditions. Some scientists also believe that stem cells derived from *cloned* human embryos, produced explicitly for such research, might prove uniquely useful for studying many genetic
diseases and devising novel therapies. Public reaction to the prospect of
cloning-for-biomedical-research has been mixed, with some Americans supporting it for its medical promise and others opposing it because it requires
the exploitation and destruction of nascent human life, which would be created solely for research purposes.

Human Cloning: What Is at Stake?

The intense attention given to human cloning in both its potential uses, for
reproduction as well as for research, strongly suggests that people do not regard it as just another new technology. Instead, we see it as something quite
different, something that touches fundamental aspects of our humanity. The
notion of cloning raises issues about identity and individuality, the meaning
of having children, the difference between procreation and manufacture, and
the relationship between the generations. It also raises new questions about
the manipulation of some human beings for the benefit of others, the freedom and value of biomedical inquiry, our obligation to heal the sick (and its
limits), and the respect and protection owed to nascent human life.

Finally, the legislative debates over human cloning raise large questions
about the relationship between science and society, especially about whether
society can or should exercise ethical and prudential control over biomedical
technology and the conduct of biomedical research. Rarely has such a seemingly small innovation raised such big questions.

The Inquiry: Our Point of Departure

As Members of the President's Council on Bioethics, we have taken up the
larger ethical and social inquiry called for in the NBAC and NAS reports,
with the aim of advancing public understanding and informing public policy

on the matter. We have attempted to consider human cloning (both for producing children and for biomedical research) within its larger human, technological, and ethical contexts, rather than to view it as an isolated technical development. We focus first on the broad human goods that it may serve as well as threaten, rather than on the immediate impact of the technique itself. By our broad approach, our starting on the plane of human goods, and our open spirit of inquiry, we hope to contribute to a richer and deeper understanding of what human cloning means, how we should think about it, and what we should do about it.

On some matters discussed in this report, Members of the Council are not of one mind. Rather than bury these differences in search of a spurious consensus, we have sought to present all views fully and fairly, while recording our agreements as well as our genuine diversity of perspectives, including our differences on the final recommendations to be made. By this means, we hope to help policymakers and the general public appreciate more thoroughly the difficulty of the issues and the competing goods that are at stake.

Fair and Accurate Terminology

There is today much confusion about the terms used to discuss human cloning, regarding both the activity involved and the entities that result. The Council stresses the importance of striving not only for accuracy but also for fairness, especially because the choice of terms can decisively affect the way questions are posed, and hence how answers are given. We have sought terminology that most accurately conveys the descriptive reality of the matter, in order that the moral arguments can then proceed on the merits. We have resisted the temptation to solve the moral questions by artful redefinition or by denying to some morally crucial element a name that makes clear that there is a moral question to be faced.

On the basis of (1) a careful analysis of the act of cloning, and its relation to the means by which it is accomplished and the purposes it may serve, and (2) an extensive critical examination of alternative terminologies, the Council has adopted the following definitions for the most important terms in the matter of human cloning:

- *Cloning*: A form of reproduction in which offspring result not from the chance union of egg and sperm (sexual reproduction) but from the deliberate replication of the genetic makeup of another single individual (asexual reproduction).

- *Human cloning*: The asexual production of a new human organism that is, at all stages of development, genetically virtually identical to a currently existing or previously existing human being. It would be accomplished by introducing the nuclear material of a human somatic cell (donor) into an oocyte (egg) whose own nucleus has been removed or inactivated, yielding a product that has a human genetic constitution virtually identical to the donor of the somatic cell. (This procedure is known as "somatic cell nuclear transfer," or SCNT). We have declined to use the terms "reproductive cloning" and "therapeutic cloning." We have chosen instead to use the following designations:

  - *Cloning-to-produce-children*: Production of a cloned human embryo, formed for the (proximate) purpose of initiating a pregnancy, with the (ultimate) goal of producing a child who will be genetically virtually identical to a currently existing or previously existing individual.

  - *Cloning-for-biomedical-research*: Production of a cloned human embryo, formed for the (proximate) purpose of using it in research or for extracting its stem cells, with the (ultimate) goals of gaining scientific knowledge of normal and abnormal development and of developing cures for human diseases.

  - *Cloned human embryo*: (a) A human embryo resulting from the nuclear transfer process (as contrasted with a human embryo arising from the union of egg and sperm). (b) The immediate (and developing) product of the initial act of cloning, accomplished by successful SCNT, whether used subsequently in attempts to produce children or in biomedical research.

Scientific Background

Cloning research and stem cell research are being actively investigated and the state of the science is changing rapidly; significant new developments could change some of the interpretations in our report. At present, however, a few general points may be highlighted.

- *The technique of cloning.* The following steps have been used to produce live offspring in the mammalian species that have been successfully cloned. Obtain an egg cell from a female of a mammalian species. Remove its nuclear DNA, to produce an enucleated egg. Insert the nucleus of a donor adult cell into the enucleated egg, to produce a reconstructed egg. Activate the reconstructed egg with chemicals or electric current, to stimulate it to commence cell division. Sustain development of the cloned embryo to a suitable stage in vitro, and then transfer it to the uterus of a female host that has been suitably prepared to receive it. Bring to live birth a cloned animal that is genetically virtually identical (except for the mitochondrial DNA) to the animal that donated the adult cell nucleus.

- *Animal cloning: low success rates, high morbidity.* At least seven species of mammals (none of them primates) have been successfully cloned to produce live births. Yet the production of live cloned offspring is rare and the failure rate is high: more than 90 percent of attempts to initiate a clonal pregnancy do not result in successful live birth. Moreover, the live-born cloned animals suffer high rates of deformity and disability, both at birth and later on. Some biologists attribute these failures to errors or incompleteness of epigenetic reprogramming of the somatic cell nucleus.

- *Attempts at human cloning.* At this writing, it is uncertain whether anyone has attempted cloning-to-produce-children (although at least one physician is now claiming to have initiated several active clonal pregnancies, and others are reportedly working on it). We do not know whether a transferred cloned human embryo can progress all the way to live birth.

- *Stem cell research.* Human embryonic stem cells have been isolated from embryos (produced by IVF) at the blastocyst stage, or from the germinal tissue of fetuses. Human adult stem (or multipotent) cells have been isolated from a variety of tissues. Such cell populations can be differentiated in vitro into a number of different cell types, and are currently being studied intensely for their possible uses in regenerative medicine. Most scientists working in the field believe that stem cells (both embryonic and adult) hold great promise as routes toward cures and treatments for many human diseases and disabilities. All stem cell research is at a very early stage, and it is too soon to tell which approaches will prove most useful, and for which purposes.

- *The transplant rejection problem.* To be effective as long-term treatments, cell transplantation therapies will have to overcome the immune rejection problem. Cells and tissues derived from *adult* stem cells and returned to the patient from whom they were taken would not be subject (at least in principle) to immune rejection.

- *Stem cells from cloned embryos.* Human embryonic stem cell preparations could potentially be produced by using somatic cell nuclear transfer to produce a cloned human embryo, and then taking it apart at the blastocyst stage and isolating stem cells. These stem cells would be genetically virtually identical to cells from the nucleus donor, and thus could potentially be of great value in biomedical research. Very little work of this sort has been done to date in animals, and there are as yet no *published* reports of cloned *human* embryos grown to the blastocyst stage. Although the promise of such research is at this time unknown, most researchers believe it will yield very useful and important knowledge, pointing toward new therapies and offering one of several possible routes to circumvent the immune rejection problem. Although some animal experimental results are indeed quite encouraging, they also demonstrate some tendency even of cloned stem cells to stimulate an immune response.
- *The fate of embryos used in research.* All extractions of stem cells from human embryos, cloned or not, involve the destruction of these embryos.

The Ethics of Cloning-to-Produce-Children

Two separate national-level reports on human cloning (NBAC 1997; NAS 2002) concluded that attempts to clone a human being would be unethical at this time due to safety concerns and the likelihood of harm to those involved. The Council concurs in this conclusion. But we have extended the work of these distinguished bodies by undertaking a broad ethical examination of the merits of, and difficulties with, cloning-to-produce-children.

Cloning-to-produce-children might serve several purposes. It might allow infertile couples or others to have genetically-related children; permit couples at risk of conceiving a child with a genetic disease to avoid having an afflicted child; allow the bearing of a child who could become an ideal transplant donor for a particular patient in need; enable a parent to keep a living connection with a dead or dying child or spouse, or even to try to "replicate" individuals of great talent or beauty. These purposes have been defended by appeals to the goods of freedom, existence (as opposed to nonexistence), and well-being—all vitally important ideals.

A major weakness in these arguments supporting cloning-to-produce-children is that they overemphasize the freedom, desires, and control of parents, and pay insufficient attention to the well-being of the cloned child-to-be. The Council holds that, once the child-to-be is carefully considered, these arguments are not sufficient to overcome the powerful case against engaging in cloning-to-produce-children.

First, cloning-to-produce-children would violate the principles of the ethics of human research. Given the high rates of morbidity and mortality in the cloning of other mammals, we believe that cloning-to-produce-children would be extremely unsafe, and that attempts to produce a cloned child would be highly unethical. Indeed, our moral analysis of this matter leads us to conclude that this is not, as is sometimes implied, a merely temporary objection, easily removed by the improvement of technique. We offer reasons for believing that the safety risks might be enduring, and offer arguments in support of a strong conclusion: that conducting experiments in an effort to make cloning-to-produce-children safer would itself be an unacceptable violation of the norms of research ethics. *There seems to be no ethical way to try to discover whether cloning-to-produce-children can become safe, now or in the future.*

If carefully considered, the concerns about safety also begin to reveal the ethical principles that should guide a broader assessment of cloning-to-produce-children: the principles of freedom, equality, and human dignity. To appreciate the broader human significance of cloning-to-produce-children, one needs first to reflect on the meaning of having children; the meaning of asexual, as opposed to sexual, reproduction; the importance of origins and genetic endowment for identity and sense of self; the meaning of exercising greater human control over the processes and "products" of human reproduction; and the difference between begetting and making. Reflecting on these topics, the Council has identified five categories of concern regarding cloning-to-produce-children. (Different Council Members give varying moral weight to these different concerns.)

- *Problems of identity and individuality*: Cloned children may experience serious problems of identity both because each will be genetically virtually identical to a human being who has already lived and because the expectations for their lives may be shadowed by constant comparisons to the life of the "original."
- *Concerns regarding manufacture*: Cloned children would be the first human beings whose entire genetic makeup is selected in advance. They might come to be considered more like products of a designed manufacturing process than "gifts" whom their parents are prepared

to accept as they are. Such an attitude toward children could also contribute to increased commercialization and industrialization of human procreation.

- *The prospect of a new eugenics*: Cloning, if successful, might serve the ends of individualized eugenic enhancement, either by avoiding the genetic defects that may arise when human reproduction is left to chance, or by preserving and perpetuating outstanding genetic traits, including the possibility, someday in the future, of using cloning to perpetuate genetically engineered enhancements.

- *Troubled family relations*: By confounding and transgressing the natural boundaries between generations, cloning could strain the social ties between them. Fathers could become "twin brothers" to their "sons"; mothers could give birth to their genetic twins; and grandparents would also be the "genetic parents" of their grandchildren. Genetic relation to only one parent might produce special difficulties for family life.

- *Effects on society*: Cloning-to-produce-children would affect not only the direct participants, but also the entire society that allows or supports this activity. Even if practiced on a small scale, it could affect the way society looks at children and set a precedent for future nontherapeutic interventions into the human genetic endowment or novel forms of control by one generation over the next. In the absence of wisdom regarding these matters, prudence dictates caution and restraint.

Conclusion: For some or all of these reasons, the Council is in full agreement that cloning-to-produce-children is not only unsafe but also morally unacceptable, and ought not to be attempted.

The Ethics of Cloning-for-Biomedical-Research

Ethical assessment of cloning-for-biomedical-research is far more vexing. On the one hand, such research could lead to important knowledge about human embryological development and gene action, both normal and abnormal, ultimately resulting in treatments and cures for many dreaded illnesses and disabilities. On the other hand, the research is controversial because it involves the deliberate production, use, and ultimate destruction of cloned human embryos, and because the cloned embryos produced for research are no different from those that could be used in attempts to produce cloned children. The difficulty is compounded by what are, for now, unanswerable questions as to whether the research will in fact yield the benefits hoped for, and whether other promising and morally nonproblematic approaches might yield comparable benefits. The Council, reflecting the differences of opinion in American society, is divided regarding the ethics of research involving (cloned) embryos. *Yet we agree that all parties to the debate have concerns vital to defend, vital not only to themselves but to all of us. No human being and no society can afford to be callous to the needs of suffering humanity, or cavalier about the treatment of nascent human life, or indifferent to the social effects of adopting one course of action rather than another.*

To make clear to all what is at stake in the decision, Council Members have presented, as strongly as possible, the competing ethical cases for and against cloning-for-biomedical-research in the form of first-person attempts at moral suasion. Each case has tried to address what is owed to suffering humanity, to the human embryo, and to the broader society. Within each case, supporters of the position in question speak only for themselves, and not for the Council as a whole.

A. The Moral Case for Cloning-for-Biomedical-Research

The moral case for proceeding with the research rests on our obligation to try to relieve human suffering, an obligation that falls most powerfully on medical practitioners and biomedical researchers. We who support cloning-for-biomedical-research all agree that it may offer uniquely useful ways of investigating and possibly treating many chronic debilitating diseases and disabilities, providing aid and relief to millions. We also believe that the moral objections to this research are outweighed by the great good that may come from it. Up to this point, we who support the research all agree. But we differ among ourselves regarding the weight of the moral objections, owing to differences about the moral status of the cloned embryo. These differences are sufficient to warrant distinguishing two different moral positions within the moral case for cloning-for-biomedical-research:

Position Number One

Most Council Members who favor cloning-for-biomedical-research do so with serious moral concerns. Speaking only for ourselves, we acknowledge the following difficulties, but think that they can be addressed by setting proper boundaries.

- *Intermediate moral status.* While we take seriously concerns about the treatment of nascent human life, we believe there are sound moral reasons for not regarding the embryo in its earliest stages as the moral equivalent of a human person. We believe the embryo has a developing and intermediate moral worth that commands our special respect, but that it is morally permissible to use early-stage cloned human embryos in important research under strict regulation.
- *Deliberate Creation for Use.* We believe that concerns over the problem of deliberate creation of cloned embryos for use in research have merit, but when properly understood should not preclude cloning-for-biomedical-research. These embryos would not be "created for destruction," but for use in the service of life and medicine. They would be destroyed in the service of a great good, and this should not be obscured.
- *Going Too Far.* We acknowledge the concern that some researchers might seek to develop cloned embryos beyond the blastocyst stage, and for those of us who believe that the cloned embryo has a developing and intermediate moral status, this is a very real worry. We approve, therefore, only of research on cloned embryos that is strictly limited to the first fourteen days of development—a point near when the primitive streak is formed and before organ differentiation occurs.
- *Other Moral Hazards.* We believe that concerns about the exploitation of women and about the risk that cloning-for-biomedical-research could lead to cloning-to-produce-children can be adequately addressed by appropriate rules and regulations. These concerns need not frighten us into abandoning an important avenue of research.

Position Number Two

A few Council Members who favor cloning-for-biomedical-research do not share all the ethical qualms expressed above. Speaking only for ourselves, we hold that this research, at least for the purposes presently contemplated, presents no special moral problems, and therefore should be endorsed with enthusiasm as a potential new means of gaining knowledge to serve humankind. Because we accord no special moral status to the early-stage cloned embryo and believe it should be treated essentially like all other human cells, we believe that the moral issues involved in this research are no different from those that accompany any biomedical research. What is required is the usual commitment to high standards for the quality of research, scientific integrity, and the need to obtain informed consent from donors of the eggs and somatic cells used in nuclear transfer.

B. The Moral Case against Cloning-for-Biomedical-Research

The moral case against cloning-for-biomedical-research acknowledges the possibility—though purely speculative at the moment—that medical benefits might come from this particular avenue of experimentation. But we believe it is morally wrong to exploit and destroy developing human life, even for good reasons, and that it is unwise to open the door to the many undesirable consequences that are likely to result from this research. We find it disquieting, even somewhat ignoble, to treat what are in fact seeds of the next generation as mere raw material for satisfying the needs of our own. Only for very serious reasons should progress toward increased knowledge and medical advances be slowed. But we believe that in this case such reasons are apparent.

- *Moral status of the cloned embryo.* We hold that the case for treating the early-stage embryo as simply the moral equivalent of all other human cells (Position Number Two, above) is simply mistaken: it denies the continuous history of human individuals from the embryonic to fetal to infant stages of existence; it misunderstands the meaning of potentiality; and it ignores the hazardous moral precedent that the routinized creation, use, and destruction of nascent human life would establish. We hold that the case for according the human embryo "intermediate and developing moral status" (Position Number One, above) is also unconvincing, for reasons both biological and moral. Attempts to ground the limited measure of respect owed to a maturing embryo in certain of its developmental features do not succeed, and the invoking of a "special respect" owed to nascent human life seems to have little or no operative meaning if cloned embryos may be created in bulk and used routinely with impunity. If from one perspective the view that the embryo seems to amount to little may invite a weakening of our respect, from another perspective its seeming insignificance should awaken in us a sense of shared humanity and a special obligation to protect it.
- *The exploitation of developing human life.* To engage in cloning-for-biomedical-research requires the irreversible crossing of a very signifi-

cant moral boundary: the creation of human life expressly and exclusively for the purpose of its use in research, research that necessarily involves its deliberate destruction. If we permit this research to proceed, we will effectively be endorsing the complete transformation of nascent human life into nothing more than a resource or a tool. Doing so would coarsen our moral sensibilities and make us a different society: one less humble toward that which we cannot fully understand, less willing to extend the boundaries of human respect ever outward, and more willing to transgress moral boundaries once it appears to be in our own interests to do so.

- *Moral harm to society.* Even those who are uncertain about the precise moral status of the human embryo have sound ethical-prudential reasons to oppose cloning-for-biomedical-research. Giving moral approval to such research risks significant moral harm to our society by (1) crossing the boundary from sexual to asexual reproduction, thus approving in principle the genetic manipulation and control of nascent human life; (2) opening the door to other moral hazards, such as cloning-to-produce-children or research on later-stage human embryos and fetuses; and (3) potentially putting the federal government in the novel and unsavory position of mandating the destruction of nascent human life. Because we are concerned not only with the fate of the cloned embryos but also with where this research will lead our society, we think prudence requires us not to engage in this research.

- *What we owe the suffering.* We are certainly not deaf to the voices of suffering patients; after all, each of us already shares or will share in the hardships of mortal life. We and our loved ones are all patients or potential patients. But we are not only patients, and easing suffering is not our only moral obligation. As much as we wish to alleviate suffering now and to leave our children a world where suffering can be more effectively relieved, we also want to leave them a world in which we and they want to live—a world that honors moral limits, that respects all life whether strong or weak, and that refuses to secure the good of some human beings by sacrificing the lives of others.

Public Policy Options

The Council recognizes the challenges and risks of moving from moral assessment to public policy. Reflections on the "social contract" between science and society highlight both the importance of scientific freedom and the need for boundaries. We note that other countries often treat human cloning in the context of a broad area of biomedical technology, at the intersection of reproductive technology, embryo research, and genetics, while the public policy debate in the United States has been considering cloning largely on its own. We recognize the special difficulty in formulating sound public policy in this area, given that the two ethically distinct matters—cloning-to-produce-children and cloning-for-biomedical-research—will be mutually affected or implicated in any attempts to legislate about either. Nevertheless, our ethical and policy analysis leads us to the conclusion that some deliberate public policy at the federal level is needed in the area of human cloning.

We reviewed the following seven possible policy options and considered their relative strengths and weaknesses: (1) Professional self-regulation but no federal legislative action ("self-regulation"); (2) A ban on cloning-to-produce-children, with neither endorsement nor restriction of cloning-for-biomedical-research ("ban plus silence"); (3) A ban on cloning-to-produce-children, with regulation of the use of cloned embryos for biomedical research ("ban plus regulation"); (4) Governmental regulation, with no legislative prohibitions ("regulation of both"); (5) A ban on all human cloning, whether to produce children or for biomedical research ("ban on both"); (6) A ban on cloning-to-produce-children, with a moratorium or temporary ban on cloning-for-biomedical-research ("ban plus moratorium"); or (7) A moratorium or temporary ban on all human cloning, whether to produce children or for biomedical research ("moratorium on both").

The Council's Policy Recommendations

Having considered the benefits and drawbacks of each of these options, and taken into account our discussions and reflections throughout this report, the Council recommends two possible policy alternatives, each supported by a portion of the Members.

Majority Recommendation:

Ten Members of the Council recommend *a ban on cloning-to-produce-children combined with a four-year moratorium on cloning-for-biomedical-research. We also call for a federal review of current and projected practices of human embryo research, pre-implantation genetic diagnosis, genetic modification of human embryos and gametes, and related matters, with a view to recommending and shaping ethically sound poli-*

cies for the entire field. Speaking only for ourselves, those of us who support this recommendation do so for some or all of the following reasons:

- By permanently banning cloning-to-produce-children, this policy gives force to the strong ethical verdict against cloning-to-produce-children, unanimous in this Council (and in Congress) and widely supported by the American people. And by enacting a four-year moratorium on the creation of cloned embryos, it establishes an additional safeguard not afforded by policies that would allow the production of cloned embryos to proceed without delay.

- It calls for and provides time for further democratic deliberation about cloning-for-biomedical research, a subject about which the nation is divided and where there remains great uncertainty. A national discourse on this subject has not yet taken place in full, and a moratorium, by making it impossible for either side to cling to the status-quo, would force both to make their full case before the public. By banning all cloning for a time, it allows us to seek moral consensus on whether or not we should cross a major moral boundary (creating nascent cloned human life solely for research) and prevents our crossing it without deliberate decision. It would afford time for scientific evidence, now sorely lacking, to be gathered—from animal models and other avenues of human research—that might give us a better sense of whether cloning-for-biomedical-research would work as promised, and whether other morally nonproblematic approaches might be available. It would promote a fuller and better-informed public debate. And it would show respect for the deep moral concerns of the large number of Americans who have serious ethical problems with this research.

- Some of us hold that cloning-for-biomedical-research can never be ethically pursued, and endorse a moratorium to enable us to continue to make our case in a democratic way. Others of us support the moratorium because it would provide the time and incentive required to develop a system of national regulation that might come into use if, at the end of the four-year period, the moratorium were not reinstated or made permanent. Such a system could not be developed overnight, and therefore even those who support the research but want it regulated should see that at the very least a pause is required. In the absence of a moratorium, few proponents of the research would have much incentive to institute an effective regulatory system. Moreover, the very

process of proposing such regulations would clarify the moral and prudential judgments involved in deciding whether and how to proceed
with this research.

- A moratorium on cloning-for-biomedical-research would enable us to
consider this activity in the larger context of research and technology
in the areas of developmental biology, embryo research, and genetics,
and to pursue a more comprehensive federal regulatory system for setting and executing policy in the entire area.

- Finally, we believe that a moratorium, rather than a lasting ban, signals
a high regard for the value of biomedical research and an enduring concern for patients and families whose suffering such research may help
alleviate. It would reaffirm the principle that science can progress while
upholding the community's moral norms, and would therefore reaffirm
the community's moral support for science and biomedical technology.

The decision before us is of great importance. Our society should take the
time to make a judgment that is well-informed, respectful of strongly held
views, and representative of the priorities and principles of the American
people. We believe this ban-plus-moratorium proposal offers the best available way to a wise and prudent policy.

This position is supported by Council Members Rebecca S. Dresser, Fran-
cis Fukuyama, Robert P. George, Mary Ann Glendon, Alfonso Gómez-Lobo,
William B. Hurlbut, Leon R. Kass, Charles Krauthammer, Paul McHugh, and
Gilbert C. Meilaender.

Minority Recommendation:

Seven Members of the Council recommend *a ban on cloning-to-produce-
children, with regulation of the use of cloned embryos for biomedical research.* Speaking only for ourselves, those of us who support this recommendation do so
for some or all of the following reasons:

- By permanently banning cloning-to-produce-children, this policy gives
force to the strong ethical verdict against cloning-to-produce-children,
unanimous in this Council (and in Congress) and widely supported by
the American people. We believe that a ban on the transfer of cloned
embryos to a woman's uterus would be a sufficient and effective legal
safeguard against the practice.

- *It approves cloning-for-biomedical-research and permits it to proceed without substantial delay.* This is the most important advantage of this proposal. The research shows great promise, and its actual value can only be determined by allowing it to go forward now. Regardless of how much time we allow it, no amount of experimentation with animal models can provide the needed understanding of *human* diseases. The special benefits from working with stem cells from *cloned* human embryos cannot be obtained using embryos obtained by IVF. We believe this research could provide relief to millions of Americans, and that the government should therefore support it, within sensible limits imposed by regulation.
- It would establish, as a condition of proceeding, the necessary regulatory protections to avoid abuses and misuses of cloned embryos. These regulations might touch on the secure handling of embryos, licensing and prior review of research projects, the protection of egg donors, and the provision of equal access to benefits.
- Some of us also believe that mechanisms to regulate cloning-for-biomedical-research should be part of a larger regulatory program governing all research involving human embryos, and that the federal government should initiate a review of present and projected practices of human embryo research, with the aim of establishing reasonable policies on the matter.

Permitting cloning-for-biomedical-research now, while governing it through a prudent and sensible regulatory regime, is the most appropriate way to allow important research to proceed while insuring that abuses are prevented. We believe that the legitimate concerns about human cloning expressed throughout this report are sufficiently addressed by this ban–plus–regulation proposal, and that the nation should affirm and support the responsible effort to find treatments and cures that might help many who are suffering.

This position is supported by Council Members Elizabeth H. Blackburn, Daniel W. Foster, Michael S. Gazzaniga, William F. May, Janet D. Rowley, Michael J. Sandel, and James Q. Wilson.

July 2002

Contributors

Gaymon Bennett is a doctoral student at the Graduate Theological Union, in Berkeley, California, and research assistant to the ethics advisory board of the Geron Corporation. He is coeditor, with Ted Peters, of *Bridging Science and Religion*.

Ronald Cole-Turner is the H. Parker Sharp Professor of Theology and Ethics at Pittsburgh Theological Seminary and an ordained minister in the United Church of Christ. Recent publications include the edited volumes, *Human Cloning: Religious Perspectives* and *Beyond Cloning: Religion and the Remaking of Humanity*.

Kevin FitzGerald holds the David P. Lauler Chair in Catholic Health Care Ethics at the Center for Clinical Bioethics and is associate professor of oncology at Georgetown University. Recent publications include "Knowledge and Wisdom: Human Genetic Interventions with Religious Insight," *St. Thomas Law Review* (summer 2001), and "Cloning: Can It Be Good for Us? An Overview of Cloning Technology and Its Moral Implications," *University of Toledo Law Review* (spring 2001).

Gene Outka is the Dwight Professor of Philosophy and Christian Ethics at Yale University. Recent publications include "The Particularist Turn in Theological and Philosophical Ethics," in Lisa Sowle Cahill and James F. Childress, eds., *Christian Ethics: Problems and Prospects* and "Theocentric Love and the Augustinian Legacy: Honoring Differences and Likenesses Between God and Ourselves," *Journal of the Society of Christian Ethics*, 22 (2002).

Ted Peters is professor of systematic theology at Pacific Lutheran Theological Seminary and the Graduate Theological Union and research scholar at the Center for Theology and the Natural Sciences. He is the author of *GOD: The World's Future* and *Playing God? Genetic Determinism and Human Freedom*.

James C. Peterson is the C. C. Dickson Professor of Theology and Ethics at Wingate University. He is the author of *Genetic Turning Points: The Ethics of Human Genetic Intervention*.

Robert Song is lecturer in Christian ethics at the University of Durham. He is the author of *Genetics: Fabricating the Future* and *Christianity and Liberal Society*.

Brent Waters is director of the Jerre L. and Mary Joy Center for Ethics and Values and associate professor of Christian social ethics at Garrett-Evangelical Theological Seminary. He is the author of *Reproductive Technology: Towards a Theology of Procreative Stewardship* and coauthor, with Ronald Cole-Turner, of *Pastoral Genetics: Theology and Care at the Beginning of Life*.

Sondra Wheeler is the Martha Ashby Carr Professor of Christian Ethics at Wesley Theological Seminary. Her most recent publications in bioethics are "Parental Liberty and the Right of Access to Germline Intervention," in Audrey R. Chapman and Mark Frankel, eds., *Human Genetic Modifications Across Generations: Assessing Scientific, Ethical, Religious and Policy Issues,* and "Contingency, Tragedy, and the Virtues of Parenting" in Ronald Cole-Turner, ed., *Beyond Cloning.*

Laurie Zoloth is professor of medical ethics and humanities at the Feinberg School of Medicine at Northwestern University. Her recent publications include *The Human Embryonic Stem Cell Debate: Science, Ethics, and Public Policy,* coedited with Suzanne Holland and Karen Lebacqz, and *Health Care and the Ethics of Encounter: A Jewish Discussion of Social Justice.*

Index